MILADY'S
STANDARD
Cosmetology
STUDY GUIDE
The Essential Companion

MILADY'S
STANDARD
Cosmetology
STUDY GUIDE
The Essential Companion

Letha Barnes
with Lisha Barnes

THOMSON ™

DELMAR LEARNING

Australia   Canada   Mexico   Singapore   Spain   United Kingdom   United States

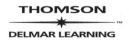

Milady's Standard:
Cosmetology Study Guide : The Essential Companion
by Letha Barnes and Lisha Barnes

NOTICE TO THE READER

Publisher does not warrant or guarantee any of the products described herein or perform any independent analysis in connection with any of the product information contained herein. Publisher does not assume, and expressly disclaims, any obligation to obtain and include information other than that provided to it by the manufacturer.

The reader is expressly warned to consider and adopt all safety precautions that might be indicated by the activities herein and to avoid all potential hazards. By following the instructions contained herein, the reader willingly assumes all risks in connection with such instructions.

The Publisher makes no representation or warranties of any kind, including but not limited to, the warranties of fitness for particular purpose or merchantability, nor are any such representations implied with respect to the material set forth herein, and the publisher takes no responsibility with respect to such material. The publisher shall not be liable for any special, consequential, or exemplary damages resulting, in whole or part, from the readers' use of, or reliance upon, this material.

Contents

CHAPTER 11
HAIRCUTTING 175

CHAPTER 12
HAIRSTYLING 191

CHAPTER 13
BRAIDING AND BRAID
EXTENSIONS 218

CHAPTER 18
HAIR REMOVAL 297

CHAPTER 19
FACIALS 308

CHAPTER 20
FACIAL MAKEUP 328

CHAPTER 21
NAIL STRUCTURE AND GROWTH . .342

Preface

Introduction

Congratulations! As a student of cosmetology you now hold in your hands one of the most essential tools available to successfully progress through your course of study. You have chosen to embark upon a career in cosmetology, which can be a life-transforming event. In that journey, you deserve the best possible education, which can be accomplished by using the best possible educational tools available. *The Essential Companion* is just such a tool.

Purpose

The purpose of *The Essential Companion* is to act as a study guide for you, the student, in achieving the objectives of each lesson presented by your instructors. Each chapter is designed to be a critical companion to the chapter you are assigned in the *Milady's Standard: Cosmetology* textbook. The study guide is designed to emphasize active, conceptual learning and to consolidate your understanding of the textbook. Information presented is provided in an informal tone, allowing the study guide to take on the role of a private tutor or companion to aid you in mastering the text content.

Design

Each chapter of *The Essential Companion* is divided into six sections as follows:

Essential Objectives

The objectives set forth for the textbook chapter are restated to help you focus on the goals for the lesson.

Essential Subject

This section provides a brief overview about why the subject matter contained in the chapter is essential in the life of a successful cosmetologist.

Essential Concepts

This section provides an outline or brief overview of the chapter content.

Essential Experiences

This section contains activities, projects, and puzzles which are designed to reinforce the content contained in the textbook chapter and increase your retention of the material studied. The Essential Experiences are designed to help you retain important information on a given subject through fun and interesting activities. The activities include personal research projects, mind mapping, windowpaning, matching exercises, crossword puzzles, word search puzzles, word scramble puzzles, role-playing, and more.

To help you understand some of the active learning exercises you will use, a brief explanation is provided here. Mind mapping is used for developing an innovative and more creative approach to thinking. It simply creates a free-flowing outline of material or information. It is easy to learn, and when you master the technique you will be able to organize an entire project or chapter in a matter of minutes. Mind mapping will allow you to release your creativity and engage both hemispheres of your brain. This technique has proved more effective than the linear form of note taking for most students. When mind mapping, the central or main idea is more clearly defined. The map lays out the relative

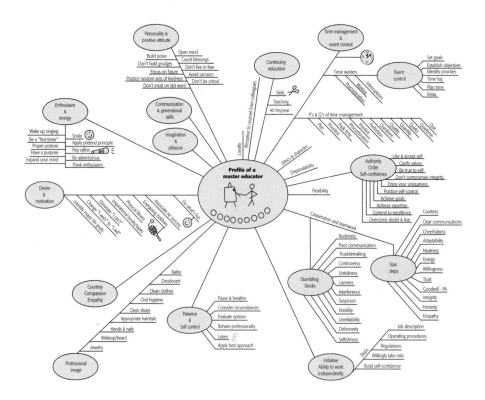

importance of each idea or element of the subject matter. For example, the more-important ideas or material will be nearer the center, and the less-important material will be located in the outer parameters. Proximity and connections are used to establish the links between key concepts or ideas. The result is that review and recall will occur more quickly and be more effective. As you develop the art of mind mapping, you will see that each one takes on a unique appearance, which even adds to your recall ability of different topics or subjects. An example of how all the qualities, skills, and characteristics of an educator could be placed in a mind map is provided below.

Windowpaning is the process of transferring key elements, points, or steps in a lesson into visual images that are then hand-sketched into the squares or "panes" of a matrix. Your mind thinks in pictures or images. Research indicates that people can retain in their short-term memory an average of seven bits of information with a variation of two on the plus or minus side. Therefore, it is recommended that you complete windowpanes with no more than nine panes for a given topic. Refer to the example of a windowpane on how to perform cardiopulmonary resuscitation (CPR).

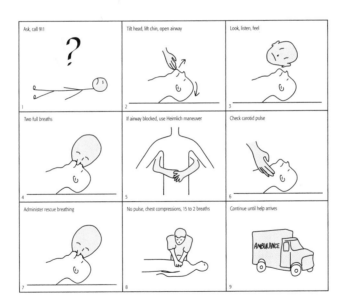

Essential Review

This section contains a quiz, which may include multiple choice or completion questions, designed to help you measure your understanding of the key concepts presented in the textbook chapter.

Essential Discoveries and Accomplishments

This section is simply your personal journal regarding the material studied. It is suggested that you jot notes about the concepts in the chapter that were the hardest for you to understand or remember. Next, consider yourself in the role of the "teacher" and think about what you would tell your students to help them *discover* and understand those difficult concepts. It is suggested that you share your **Essential Discoveries** with other students in your class and to determine if what you have discovered is also beneficial to them. As a result of feedback from other students, you may want to revise your journal and include some of the good ideas received from your peers. Under "Accomplishments," list at least three things you have accomplished since your last entry that relate to your career goals.

You may find it helpful to read the Essential Subject and Essential Concepts found in the study guide before reading the actual chapter in the textbook. Upon completion of the chapter, you will then want to complete the Essential Experiences, Essential Discoveries and Accomplishments, and Essential Review.

By choosing an institution which utilizes educational materials published by Milady Thomson Learning, the industry leader in cosmetology education and technology, you have taken a significant step toward a rewarding and successful career. You have chosen proven performance and longevity by choosing Milady. You have chosen wisely as well. May success and good fortune accompany you in every step you take with *Milady's Standard: Cosmetology* and *The Essential Companion.* We believe that with the right tools, your commitment to the best education possible, and your passion for an exciting industry, you will experience all the joys and rewards possible in a great career!

Best wishes for success!

Letha Barnes, Director,
The Career Institute,
Milady Thomson Learning

Acknowledgments

My thanks to the staff and students of Olympian University of Cosmetology, especially Field Administrator Lisha Barnes and instructors Tammy Hingtgen, Maggie Biancaniello, and Melissa Stevenson, who have provided input, ideas, feedback, and encouragement for this project. Their support and loyalty are greatly appreciated.

chapter 1

Cosmetology: The History and Opportunities

essential objectives

After studying this chapter and completing the Essential Companion *components, you should be able to:*

1. Describe the early origins of hairstyling and barbering.

2. Name some of the pioneers of modern cosmetology and their role in its development.

3. Describe the advancements made in cosmetology during the nineteenth and twentieth centuries.

4. List the career opportunities available to a licensed cosmetologist.

essential history and opportunities

Why is knowing about this history and evolution of this industry so important to my success in cosmetology or a related field?

As a professional in this industry, your overall knowledge about the field in general will impact your credibility with your clients and help you serve them better. A study of the trends throughout history will also establish that many repeat themselves over time. Thus, the more you know about the history of cosmetology, the more prepared you will be for the changing trends throughout your career.

As indicated in your text, society as a whole now has access to professional hair, skin, and nail care services. Therefore, it is important for you to know about all the various career paths available to you in order to determine which one best suits you.

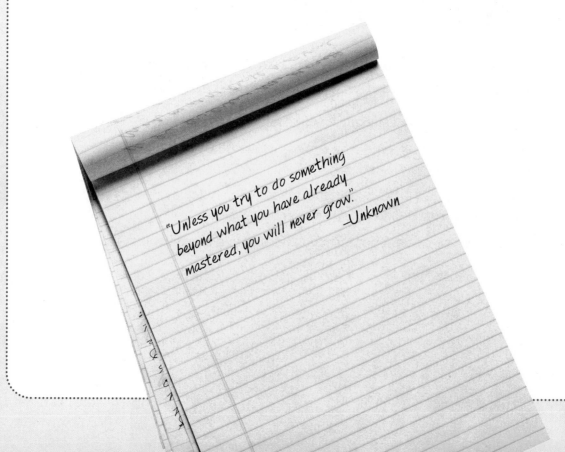

"Unless you try to do something beyond what you have already mastered, you will never grow."
—Unknown

essential concepts

What are the essentials about the industry's history and the career opportunities available?

Nearly every society has found it necessary to confine, cut, or manage the hair in order to keep it out of the way. The human species has always had a basic desire to look good. As we look at history, that desire for personal adornment has varied in form from the ornately curled, blonde wigs of Roman matrons to the sleek, waved haircuts of the flappers in the 1920s.

In preindustrial societies, hairstyling was used to indicate a person's social status. For example, primitive men would fasten bones, feathers, and other items into their hair for the purpose of impressing the lowly and frightening the enemy with their rank and prowess. Caesar made the noblemen of the ancient Gauls cut off their hair as a sign of submission when he conquered them. In addition, occupations have been indicated by hair over history, such as the gray wigs worn by the barristers (lawyers) of England and the lacquered black wigs worn by Japanese geishas.

Hair arrangement has also been used to indicate age or marital status. Adolescent Hindu boys shaved their heads, and boys in ancient Greece simply cut their hair. Until the twentieth century, generally only the upper classes enjoyed fashionable hairstyles. However, in the first half of the twentieth century nearly all classes of women followed the trend set by film stars like Jean Harlow or Marilyn Monroe.

Because of the general increase in wealth, the improvements in mass communication, greater individualism, and an overall attitude of informality, men and women of all classes can choose the style and color of hair that suits their interests, needs, and image. This change in perspective has greatly increased the demand for the services of licensed professionals in the cosmetology industry.

essential
1 experience

Historical Time Line

Using the material contained in the textbook and any other resources available to you, create a visual time line of hairdressing from the beginning of recorded history to the present. The top of the line will indicate the year, decade, or century, and the bottom of the time line will contain drawings or pictures (cut and pasted) of hairstyles or tools and implements that represent that era.

Use large poster board, colored markers, and any other items you can think of to re-create the history of hairdressing in a colorful and interesting manner.

The Glacial Age	Haircutting and styling were practiced; implements were shaped from sharpened flints, oyster shells, or bone; animal strips of hide were used to tie hair back or as adornment.
4000 B.C.	Ancient Egyptians used cosmetics for personal beautification, religious ceremonies, and burial ceremonies.
3000 B.C.	Nail care was recorded in Egypt and China. Egyptian men and women of high social rank wore red-orange henna on their nails; kings and queens wore deep red; lower rank wore only pale colors. The Chinese wore nails painted black or red.
1500 B.C.	Henna was used as hair dye.
500 B.C.	Golden Age of Greece; hairstyling became a highly developed art.
300 B.C.	Hairstyling was introduced in Rome; women use haircolor to indicate class—noblewomen tinted their hair red; middle-class colored their hair blonde; poor women colored their hair black.
Medieval times	(Medieval times or Middle Ages were considered to occur from approximately 500 A.D. to approximately 1400 A.D.) Cosmetology and medicine were taught as combined subjects in English universities.

essential
experience *continued*
1

Fourteenth century A.D.	Transition in Western civilization from medieval times to modern history.
Renaissance	(Began in the fourteenth century and lasted into the seventeenth century). Particular emphasis was placed on physical appearance. Hair was carefully dressed and ornaments and headdresses were worn.
1450	Barbering and surgery was separated by law.
1541	Henry VIII reunited barbers and surgeons of London by granting a charter to the Company of Barber Surgeons.
1867	Sarah Breedlove was born to former slaves.
1890	Sarah Breedlove suffered from a scalp condition and began losing her hair. She started experimenting with store-bought products and homemade remedies.
1875	Frenchman Marcel Grateau invented the technique using irons for waving and curling hair. This practice developed into the art of thermal waving, which is still known today as Marcel waving.
1890	The first hairdressing academy was opened in Chicago by a pair of Frenchmen, Brisbois and Federmeyer.
1892	Frenchman Alexandre F. Godefroy invented the hot-blast hair dryer.
1905	Charles Nessler invented the first electric perm machine.
1906	Sarah Breedlove married her third husband, C. J. Walker, and was henceforth known as Madam C. J. Walker. She began to sell her scalp conditioning and healing formula, called Madam C. J. Walker's Wonderful Hair Grower.
1910	Madam C. J. Walker moved her company to Indianapolis, where she built a factory, a hair salon, and a training school.

essential
experience *continued*

1917   Madam C. J. Walker organized a convention for her Madam C. J. Walker Hair Culturists Union of America.

1931   The preheat method of perming was introduced. Hair was wrapped using a croquignole method, and then preheated clamps were placed over the wound curls.

1932   Ralph L. Evans and Everett G. McDonough pioneered a method that used external heat generated by chemical reaction. Small flexible pads containing a chemical mixture were wound around hair strands. When pads were moistened with water, a chemical heat was released that created long-lasting curls. This was the first machineless perm.

1941   Scientists developed another method of permanent waving that used waving lotion, but did not use heat. It was called a cold wave and virtually replaced all predecessors and competitors. The terms *cold waving* and *permanent waving* almost became synonymous.

1950   Growth and expansion occurred which were unrivaled by any other time in history. Advancements in technology and innovative haircutting, chemical services, esthetics, and nail extensions occurred. (Examples include haircutting clippers, edgers, facial machines, day spas, acrylic nails and fiberglass tips, permanent makeup, artificial eyelashes, and so on.

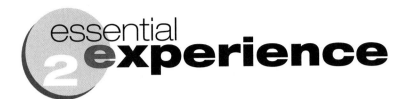

essential 2 experience

Character Study and Report

Using the library, the Internet, or other resources, further research the life of Madam C. J. Walker. Create an illustrated essay reporting how her life impacted the history of the United States as well as the history of cosmetology.

essential 3 experience

Mind Map

Mind mapping simply creates a free-flowing outline of material or information with the central or key point being located in the center. (Refer to the Preface for more details on how to create a mind map). The key point of this mind map is you as a licensed cosmetologist. Diagram the different career opportunities awaiting you upon your completion of the cosmetology course. Identify the different disciplines and branch of each of the different positions that may be obtained in that field. Use terms, pictures, and symbols as desired. Using color will increase the mind's retention and memory of the information. Keep your mind open and uncluttered and don't worry about where a line or word should go. The organization of the map will usually take care of itself.

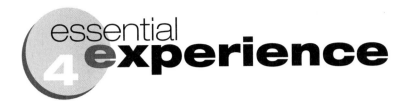

essential
4 experience

Character Study and Report

Select a twentieth-century industry icon (such as Vidal Sassoon or John Paul DeJoria) and conduct research on his or her life and career in cosmetology. Again, use the library, the Internet, trade magazines, or other resources to obtain your information. Explain the impact this person has had on the industry and why or why not he/she should be respected within the industry. Don't limit yourself to a written report. Feel free to use illustrations, photos, drawings, diagrams, and color to enhance your report and make it more meaningful.

essential
5 experience

What Does the Future Hold?

Select another student as a partner and brainstorm about where you see the future of cosmetology heading. Consider the aging of society, changing lifestyles, increasing incomes, the varying interests of men and women, and the attitudes of the young people today. Think about the styles of the future and how they will be achieved. As a team, create a poster that depicts your predictions for the future (at least into the second decade of the twenty-first century).

essential
experience
6

Word Search—Career Opportunities

After determining the correct words from the clues provided, locate the terms in the word search puzzle.

Word	Clue
_____	One who serves in a regulatory capacity
_____	One who creates new products through research and experimentation
_____	One who is licensed to practice all phases of cosmetology
_____	One who teaches
_____	One who specializes in the health and beauty of the skin
_____	One who specializes in formulating haircolor
_____	One who applies cosmetics to enhance the client's appearance
_____	One who specializes in manicuring, pedicuring, and advanced nail techniques
_____	One who demonstrates current trends, techniques, and/or products on stage
_____	One who sells products
_____	One who possesses sound business skills, including purchasing, personnel development, advertising, sales, budgeting, and people skills
_____	One who is responsible for paying bills, payroll, taxes, and the overall bottom line of the salon
_____	One who directs the creation of the right fashion look for magazines, book layouts, and other productions
_____	One who cuts and styles hair
_____	One who writes articles, books, brochures, columns, educational textbooks, and video scripts

```
B  O  A  R  D  M  E  M  B  E  R  K  M  T  T  S
S  T  E  S  T  H  E  T  I  C  I  A  N  S  S  T
A  S  D  T  T  R  E  T  T  A  M  O  I  I  I  Y
L  I  U  Y  B  Y  T  M  P  O  W  M  E  T  R  L
O  T  C  L  O  I  L  S  U  B  E  O  C  R  O  E
N  R  A  I  D  P  C  K  I  H  J  Q  U  A  L  S
M  A  T  S  W  O  H  S  C  M  S  Q  L  M  O  D
A  P  O  T  O  R  C  C  I  H  E  I  E  R  C  I
N  U  R  E  T  A  I  L  E  R  D  H  O  O  R  R
A  E  O  M  X  T  D  T  T  I  I  S  T  F  I  E
G  K  I  T  E  L  O  S  E  P  C  I  S  T  A  C
E  A  S  M  E  T  O  L  O  R  I  S  T  A  H  T
R  M  S  A  L  O  N  O  W  N  E  R  J  L  E  O
T  O  K  E  U  P  R  A  T  S  I  T  N  P  T  R
C  N  A  I  C  I  N  H  C  E  T  L  I  A  N  I
C  O  S  M  E  T  O  L  O  G  I  S  T  L  E  J
```

essential
7 experience

Scrambled Terms

Using the clues provided, unscramble the terms below.

Scramble	Correct Word
ahrsa evolbrdee	_ _ . _ _ _ _ _ _ _ _ _ _ _ _ _ _ _ *Clue:* She later became Madam C. J. Walker
raabb	_ _ _ _ _ _ *Clue:* The beard or hair of the beard
etaruga	_ _ _ _ _ _ _ _ *Clue:* He invented the marcel iron
gyoerfod	_ _ _ _ _ _ _ _ _ *Clue:* He invented the hot-blast hair dryer
ismaa	_ _ _ _ _ *Clue:* These warriors used braiding extensively to denote tribal status
laanelik	_ _ _ _ _ _ _ _ *Clue:* Another term used to denote cold wave
liarps	_ _ _ _ _ _ _ *Clue:* Wrapped from the scalp to the ends
ltegniotdolb	_ _ _ _ _ _ _ _ _ _ _ _ *Clue:* An ancient medical procedure
nhena	_ _ _ _ _ *Clue:* Extracted from the leaves of an ornamental shrub
selrahc relsens	_ _ _ _ _ _ _ _ _ _ _ _ _ _ *Clue:* He invented the electric perm machine
pass	_ _ _ _ *Clue:* They offer hair, esthetics, and specialized services
pmaytraaehor	_ _ _ _ _ _ _ _ _ _ _ _ *Clue:* The use of fragrances to induce relaxation

essential

7 experience *continued*

Scramble	Correct Word
qerlongiuoc	_ _ _ _ _ _ _ _ _ _ _ *Clue:* Wrapped from the ends to the scalp
lhpra vensa	_ _ _ _ _ _ _ _ _ _ _ _ *Clue:* A chemist
siisobrb	_ _ _ _ _ _ _ _ *Clue:* Opened the first hairdressing academy in the United States
skokeoitms	_ _ _ _ _ _ _ _ _ *Clue:* Greek meaning "skilled in the use of cosmetics"
yereemferd	_ _ _ _ _ _ _ _ _ _ *Clue:* Opened the first hairdressing academy in the United States

essential review

Using the following words, fill in the blanks below to form a thorough review of Chapter 1, "Cosmetology: The History and Opportunities."

1905	cosmetic chemist	lacquered	salon manager
1931	cosmetology	leader	salon owner
1932	curl	leaves	session hairstylist
1941	dentistry	lime	stone
$100 million	design team	lips	styles director
$50 billion	member	mentor	surgery
attitude	desire	mud	texture
bloodletting	educators	platform artist	tree bark
board member	esthetician	Pope Alexander	trends
bulk	fastest-growing	processes	washerwoman
chemicals	fourteenth	product educators	weaving
classes	glacial	professions	writer
competition	Henry VIII	pulling teeth	
champion	irons	rods	

1. It is important to continue your education throughout your career because of the constant changes to _____ , techniques, products and information.

2. Hairstyling and barbering have evolved over the centuries as one of the oldest _____ , in the world.

3. The art and science of beautifying and improving the skin, nails, and hair, and the study of cosmetics and their application, is known as _____.

4. Archeological studies reveal that haircutting and hairstyling were practiced in some form as early as the _____ age.

5. Ancient records show that coloring matter made from berries, _____ , minerals, insects, nuts, herbs, leaves, and other materials were used on the hair, skin, and nails.

6. Roman women were known to apply a mixture of _____ to their hair which was wrapped around crudely made wooden rollers to bake in the sun, creating a temporary wave.

7. Military commanders in Egypt, Babylon, and early Rome would spend hours before battle having their hair _____ and curled and their nails painted the same shade as their _____.

essential review *continued*

8. The ancient Britons brightened their blonde hair with washes made of tallow, _____ , and the extracts of certain vegetables.

9. Barbers figured prominently in the development of _____ as a recognized branch of medical practice.

10. For centuries, _____ was performed by barbers, and for more than a thousand years they were known as barber–surgeons.

11. The barber pole has its roots in the medical procedure known as _____ .

12. The _____ century marked the transition in Western civilization from medieval times to modern history.

13. _____ reunited the barbers and surgeons of London by granting a charter to the Company of Barber Surgeons.

14. In 1875, a Frenchman named Marcel Grateau developed a technique of using _____ for waving and curling the hair.

15. Beginning with the twentieth century, hairstyling began to follow trends and soon became available to all _____ of people.

16. One of the most notable success stories in the cosmetology industry is that of Madam C. J. Walker, who transformed herself from an uneducated _____ into one of the twentieth century's most successful entrepreneurs.

17. In _____ , Charles Nessler invented the electric perm machine.

18. In _____ , the preheat method was introduced, which used preheated clamps on the wound hair.

19. In 1932, the first perm method using _____ was introduced.

20. In _____ , scientists developed another method of permanent waving that used waving lotion, called a cold wave.

21. As you advance in your career as a stylist, your responsibilities may grow to include being a _____ to a younger stylist or student.

22. A color technician or haircolorist selects the best color, formulates it, and _____ it to enhance the client's hair.

23. By specializing in chemical texture services, you can give the client the look he or she wants simply by adding or removing _____ in varying degrees.

24. As a specialist in hair extensions or wig services, you can create either subtle or dramatic changes in hair length, texture, and color by adding extensions through braiding, _____, bonding, gluing, or sewing.

25. As a/an _____ , you will offer treatments to perfect the look and health of the skin.

essential review *continued*

26. If you choose to specialize in nails, you will be joining one of the _____ areas of the cosmetology profession.

27. The _____ leads by example and is responsible for helping team members achieve their goals through training, development, counseling, and coaching.

28. If you are a _____, you are responsible for paying bills, payroll, and taxes.

29. _____ are usually based out of local supply houses and travel to specific regional territories, selling professional products to licensees and establishment owners.

30. As a _____, you may consider applying for an internship with the company of your choice to study new products.

31. A _____ works to style hair and apply makeup for models being photographed for magazines, books, and other productions.

32. A _____ must be good at meeting deadlines, working within a budget, managing people, and must also have an artistic and creative flair.

33. As a _____, you will work on a team to create presentations for fashion shows, runway work, conventions, galas, or hair shows.

34. As a _____, you will travel to local, state, or national hair shows to demonstrate the most current trends, techniques, and/or products from the stage.

35. As a _____, you must have dedication, good work habits, and excellent skills to enter the honored realm that holds so many rewards.

36. _____ must have patience, people skills, communication skills, energy, and a mastery of their subject matter.

37. As a _____ with a cosmetology license, you can work for a publishing company, freelance, review new textbooks and products, or write articles, brochures, columns, educational textbooks, and video scripts.

38. Serving as a _____ on one of the various regulatory agencies in our industry allows you to take a proactive role in its growth and improvement.

39. The salon industry grosses approximately _____ per year in revenue.

40. The license you obtain upon completion of your basic course of study unlocks the door to your future, but it is our continued education and your personal _____ for success that will really launch your career.

essential
discoveries and
accomplishments

In the space below, jot some notes about the concepts in this chapter that were the hardest for you to understand or remember. Imagine finding yourself suddenly in the role of teacher and consider what you would tell your students about these difficult concepts.

Share your *Essential Discoveries* with some of the other students in your class and ask if they are helpful to them. You may want to revise your notes based on good ideas shared by your peers.

_____

_____

_____

_____

_____

_____

_____

_____

_____

_____

_____

_____

_____

_____

Life Skills

essential objectives

After studying this chapter and completing the Essential Companion *components, you should be able to:*

1. List the principles that contribute to personal and professional success.

2. Explain the concept of self-management.

3. Create a personal mission statement.

4. Explain how to set long- and short-term goals.

5. Discuss the most effective ways to manage time.

6. Describe good study habits.

7. Define *ethics*.

8. List the characteristics of a healthy, positive attitude.

essential life skills

Why do I need to learn about life skills in order to be successful as a cosmetologist?

Life skills are essential for increasing your effectiveness, your career success, and your satisfaction in your personal life as well as on the job. You may be able to achieve the highest quality technical skills, but if you are unable to manage the "big picture" of your life in general, those technical skills will yield little or no results. For example, research shows that stress has reached epidemic proportions in the United States and is having a negative impact on all of society, especially in the workplace (even in the field of cosmetology). Our goal in this chapter is to provide ideas, tools, and the best practices that you can use to increase your effectiveness, enhance your career, and feel more fulfilled with your life in general.

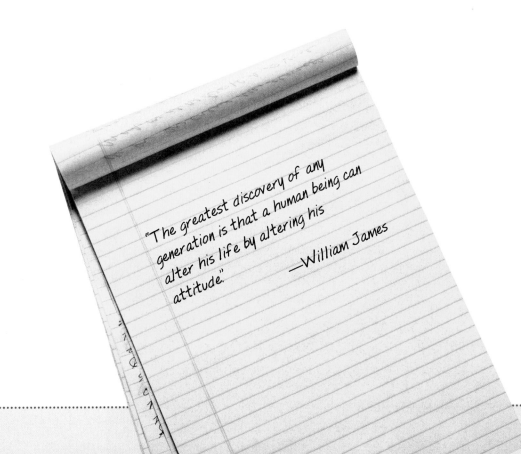

"The greatest discovery of any generation is that a human being can alter his life by altering his attitude."

—William James

essential concepts of life skills management

What do I need to know about life skills management in order to be effective as a licensed professional?

Managing your life skills requires a number of qualities, characteristics, and skills. In addition to all the technical skills you will need to master for your new career, you will need to practice general principles that form the foundation for both personal and business success. You will need to understand personal motivation and what is meant by self-management.

You will develop skills useful in expanding your creativity. Yale psychologist Robert Sternberg argues that successful intelligence goes beyond cognitive intelligence to include what he calls creative and practical intelligence. He says that people with creative intelligence know how to leverage their cognitive intelligence by *applying* what they learn in *new* and *creative* ways. This chapter introduces you to some strategies that will help you do just that. Goal setting is an integral part of any successful person's career. Thus, you need to learn how to set goals, monitor them, and expand them throughout your journey.

All of these life skills will be better managed if you also learn how to manage the events in your life. By event control, we really mean what has long been referred to as time management. Tips from the experts on time management will be useful in planning your personal quest for success.

You are now enrolled in a career program of study. Therefore, you will need to ensure that your personal study skills are up to speed and adequate to see you successfully through the course. You will even need to identify your own personal learning style in order to maximize the time spent in both study and in the classroom.

You will realize after completion of this chapter that other key ingredients to success are affected by your personality, your attitude, your approach to professional ethics,

essential concepts of life skills management

continued

and, possibly more than anything else, your ability to interact effectively with others, which is also known as human relations. Your future will be much richer if you look at your training as the opportunity to learn to manage your life in the same manner as those successful professionals who have attained many of the goals you aspire to achieve.

essential
experience
1

Goals Setting

If you have not already done so, make a chart of your short- and long-term goals as well as your action plan for achievement of those goals in the space provided. Your action plan should include the education you need to attain as well as target dates for completion. Remember, a goal is anything you can *have, be,* or *do.* For most people, goals are divided into several categories including: Career/Job, Salary/Earnings, Personal/Family Relationship, Health/Weight, Education/Skills, Knowledge, Free-Personal Time, Travel, Financial/Material Assets, Home, Transportation, and Spirituality. (Make your own chart if more space is needed).

Short-Term Goals Less than 1 Year	Action Plan/ Education Required
Long-Term Goals 1 to 10 Years	

essential 2 experience

Collage of Goals

It is a well-known belief that in order to obtain goals, we need to visualize ourselves as having already attained them. Therefore, we should picture ourselves at that desired weight, or driving that fancy sports car that appeals to us, or living in that special home we want. With that in mind, and referring back to the goals you set for yourself in Essential Experience #1, create a collage that depicts you having attained that success. For example, if you have a special home in mind, cut out a picture that represents that dream and paste it on a poster board. If you have a goal of driving a Jaguar, find a picture of a Jaguar in a magazine, cut it out, and park it in front of the house. Cut out a picture of yourself as well and place it in the Jag!

If you dream of having a wonderful spouse and two children, cut out a picture of that significant other, two children, and yourself and place them in front of the house as well. Perhaps you will have a picture of a successful platform artist performing on stage with your head overlaid on the body! Get the idea? Once you have completed the collage that holds all your dreams and goals, place it in a prominent place in your life where you will see it each and every day. By seeing yourself in those circumstances, your subconscious works even harder to help you accomplish the activities set out in your action plan so you can finally reach your goals.

essential
experience
3

Mind Map of Yourself Today

Mind mapping simply creates a free-flowing outline of material or information with the central or key point being located in the center. (Refer to the Preface for more details on how to create a mind map.) The key point of this mind map is you, as a student. Diagram the different aspects of your life as they exist today. Use terms, pictures, and symbols as desired. Using color will increase your mind's retention and memory of the information. Keep your mind open and uncluttered and don't worry about where a line or word should go. The organization of the map will usually take care of itself.

For example, draw a picture of yourself in a circle in the middle of the page. Draw a line out from the center and insert another circle where you write "student." Off the student circle, you will draw lines that might say things like: "Attend class," "study," "work with clients," and so on. Another line from the center circle might say "Mom" or "Dad" (if you are a parent), and the lines off that circle might reflect your role as a parent with tasks like "drive car pool," "coach little league," and so on. Consider all the aspects of your life and put them into the mind map in the space provided.

essential
4 experience

Mind Map Your Future

Using the collage you created in Essential Experience #2, create another mind map using the guidelines presented in the previous exercise. This time, however, draw the map as you see yourself in ten years. Upon completion of these drawings, place them in a safe place for reflection later. You may want to review these drawings at the end of your course, and then again as each new year arrives, until you reach the time you had scheduled to reach those goals you defined in Essential Experience #1.

essential experience 5

Track Your Attendance

Managing your life skills also includes something called impulse management. In this context, impulses are defined as anything that isn't an integral part of your goals; in fact, they may actually interfere with the accomplishment of your goals. According to Webster's, a goal is defined as an end that one strives to attain. An impulse is defined as a sudden inclination to act. History indicates that students often act on impulse when they decide to not attend school as scheduled. With that in mind, consider tracking your attendance, one month at a time, using the following form. This will give you clear, firsthand documentation if you are committed to achieving your goals or you are letting impulse management rule your life.

Date	Hours Missed	Reason for Absence	If Action was Impulse Management, What Actions will Prevent the Absence in the Future?

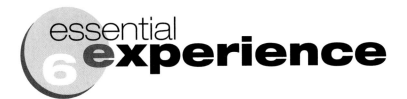

essential experience 6

Self-Assessment of Personal Characteristics

Consider the qualities and characteristics you now possess and list them either as strengths or weaknesses in the space provided. If the characteristic is a strength, state the benefits received from it. If the characteristic is a weakness, identify steps you can take to improve. Refer to the example to get started.

Strength	Benefit	Weakness	Action Plan
Promptness	Maximum use of my time; respect from others	Tardiness	Get up earlier; implement better time management strategies; be more conscious and respectful of those who are expecting me on time

essential
7 experience

Time Management

For one week, track your time in thirty-minute increments. While this may seem like a drudgery and cause you to groan, you will find the results totally enlightening! Take a look at how much time you spent in class, how much time you spent (or didn't spend) studying, how much time you spent eating and sleeping, how much quality time you spent with your family, how much time you lost on unimportant activities, and so on.

Time Utilization Log

Time	Sun	Mon	Tues	Wed	Thu	Fri	Sat
7:00 A.M.							
7:30 A.M.							
8:00 A.M.							
8:30 A.M.							
9:00 A.M.							
9:30 A.M.							
10:00 A.M.							
10:30 A.M.							
11:00 A.M.							
11:30 A.M.							
12:00 P.M.							
12:30 P.M.							
1:00 P.M.							
1:30 P.M.							
2:00 P.M.							
2:30 P.M.							
3:00 P.M.							
3:30 P.M.							
4:00 P.M.							
4:30 P.M.							
5:00 P.M.							
5:30 P.M.							
6:00 P.M.							
6:30 P.M.							
7:00 P.M.							
7:30 P.M.							
8:00 P.M.							
8:30 P.M.							
9:00 P.M.							
9:30 P.M.							
10:00 P.M.							
10:30 P.M.							
11:00 P.M.							

essential
experience
8

Action Plan for Time Management

After you have analyzed the time utilization log thoroughly, develop a personal action plan (using the chart below) for managing your time in the following week better. To help you do that, you need to identify the activities you wish to complete in the next seven days. You then need to prioritize those activities as A—greatest importance; B—average importance; C—least importance. As you progress through the week, indicate when each of the tasks has been completed.

Priorites for the Current Week		
Activities to Complete	**Priority Rank**	**Date Completed**

essential
experience
9

Is Your Bad Attitude an Addiction?

Experts tell us that the first step in addressing any addiction is recognizing, defining, and admitting the problem. Definitions: **Addict**—to habitually or obsessively devote or surrender (oneself) to something. **Addiction**—the compulsive need for (or dependence on) and use of a habit-forming substance (or behavior) characterized by tolerance and by well-defined physiological symptoms upon withdrawal. **Dependence**—the quality or state of being subordinate to something else. Please answer the following questions as honestly as you can.

1. Do you lose productive time due to your bad attitude? ___ Yes ___ No

2. Is your bad attitude making your home life unhappy? ___ Yes ___ No

3. Have you ever felt remorse because of your bad attitude? ___ Yes ___ No

4. Have you gotten into financial difficulties because of your bad attitude? ___ Yes ___ No

5. Do you turn to lower companions and an inferior environment because of your bad attitude? ___ Yes ___ No

6. Does your bad attitude make you careless with your family's welfare? ___ Yes ___ No

7. Has your ambition decreased because of your bad attitude? ___ Yes ___ No

8. Does your bad attitude cause your difficulty in sleeping? ___ Yes ___ No

9. Has your efficiency ever decreased because of your bad attitude? ___ Yes ___ No

10. Is your bad attitude jeopardizing your job or business? ___ Yes ___ No

11. Do you use your bad attitude to escape from worries or troubles? ___ Yes ___ No

12. Have you ever experienced memory loss due to your bad attitude? ___ Yes ___ No

13. Has your supervisor ever counseled you because of your bad attitude? ___ Yes ___ No

14. Is your bad attitude an absolute must in your daily life? ___ Yes ___ No

essential
experience *continued*

9

15. Have you ever been to a hospital or institution because of your
bad attitude?   ___ Yes   ___ No

If you have answered "yes" to any ONE of these questions, this is a definite WARNING that
you may be dependent upon your bad attitude.

If you answered "yes" to any TWO of these questions, the chances that you are dependent
on your bad attitude are high.

If you answered "yes" to THREE or more, you definitely are dependent upon your bad
attitude.

To begin immediate recovery from this dependency, SMILE, think positive thoughts, speak
positive self-affirmations, and visualize personal health, happiness, and success!

Questions adapted from Johns Hopkins University Hospital.

essential review

Using the following words, fill in the blanks below to form a thorough review of Chapter 2, "Life Skills."

Words or terms may be used more than once.

accomplishment	disregard	persistent	rules
attitude	energy	personality	self-confidence
bathe	free	philosophies	self-esteem
busy	goals	prescription	social
caring	hope	prioritized	strengths
clothing	human relations	problem-solve	success
communicate	interactive	procrastination	systematic
cry	intuitive	professional	technical
customer service	laugh	professional image	temperature
deportment	licensee	psychological	time-out
desire	mature adult	punctuality	values
details	motivation	reader/listener	visualize
diplomacy	passion	respect	vocabulary
discipline	perceive	reward	weaknesses

1. Your _____ skills need to rest on a solid foundation of life skills.

2. Life skills are a set of tools and guidelines that prepare you for living as a _____ in a complicated world.

3. One important life skill is that of being genuinely _____ and helpful to other people.

4. Another necessary life skill is that of maintaining a cooperative _____ in all situations.

5. The way you act toward others and handle yourself will determine whether you can sustain _____ .

6. You can have all the talent in the world and still not be successful if your talent is not fueled by the _____ for your work that will sustain you over the course of your career.

7. _____ is based on inner strength and begins with trusting your ability to reach your goals.

8. The more you _____ yourself as a success, the more easily it is to turn your goals into realities.

essential review *continued*

9. Principles or guidelines for helping you achieve success include building on your _____, being kind to yourself, defining success as you see it, practicing new behaviors, and separating your personal life from your work.

10. Successful people make a point of relating to everyone they know with a conscious feeling of _____.

11. _____ robs you of self-esteem.

12. The best _____ for learning comes from an inner desire to know.

13. For most people, basic human needs are arranged in the following order: physical, emotional, _____ , mental, and spiritual.

14. To enhance skill creativity, you should stop criticizing yourself, stop asking others what to do, change your _____ , and not try to go it totally alone.

15. A personal mission statement sets forth the _____ you plan to live by and establishes future goals.

16. Unsuccessful people have no motivation, no _____ , or no plan of action for attaining goals.

17. The most successful professionals continue to set new _____ for themselves, even those who have accumulated fame, fortune, and respect.

18. To manage time more effectively, tasks should be _____, which means making a list of tasks that need to be done in the order of most to least important.

19. Give yourself a _____ whenever you are frustrated, overwhelmed, irritated, worried, or feeling guilty about something.

20. Schedule at least one block of _____ time each day.

21. It is vitally important to be able to apply what you have been taught, and there is no way to do that except by bringing a sense of _____ to your studies.

22. _____ learners appreciate instructors who can involve them in the learning experience and who are supportive, sympathetic, and friendly.

23. Reader/listener learners are eager to find the reasons for things and are excellent at remembering facts and _____ .

24. _____ learners study best by themselves because they can concentrate better.

25. To study effectively, you must be _____, disciplined, and stay focused on your reason for studying—keeping your goals in mind.

26. Ethics are the principles of good character, proper conduct, and moral judgment, expressed through personality, _____ skills, and professional image.

essential review *continued*

27. The most ethical people make a commitment to cultivating the character traits of honesty, compassion, attentiveness, _____, cooperativeness, an agreeable personality, self-care, integrity, discretion, and clear communication.

28. Your _____ is the sum total of who you are and it is what distinguishes you from another person.

29. Ingredients for a healthy, well-developed attitude include _____, soft tone of voice, emotional stability, sensitivity, high values and goals, receptivity, and communication skills.

30. The ability to understand people is the key to operating effectively in cosmetology because _____ is central to success.

31. Effective ways for handling the ups and downs of human relations include responding instead of reacting, believing in yourself, talking less and listening more, being attentive, and taking your own _____.

32. One of the Golden Rules of Human Relations is to communicate from your heart and _____ from your head.

33. Another Golden Rule of Human Relations is to _____ often.

essential discoveries and accomplishments

In the space below, jot some notes about what concepts of this chapter were hardest for you to understand or remember. Imagine finding yourself suddenly in the role of teacher and consider what you would tell your students about these difficult concepts.

Share your *Essential Discoveries* with some of the other students in your class and ask if they are helpful to them. You may want to revise your notes based on good ideas shared by your peers. Under "Accomplishments," list at least three things you have accomplished since your last entry that relate to your career goals.

Discoveries:

_____

_____

_____

_____

_____

Accomplishments:

_____

_____

_____

_____

_____

_____

Your Professional Image

essential objectives

After studying this chapter and completing the Essential Companion *components, you should be able to:*

1. Define professional image.

2. Explain the concept of wellness as it relates to image.

3. List the three basic habits of daily personal hygiene.

4. Explain the concept of dressing for success.

5. Describe methods for achieving balance and reducing stress.

6. Identify the basic principles of sound nutrition, sleep, and exercise.

7. Demonstrate ways to improve posture, both standing and sitting.

8. Demonstrate an understanding of ergonomic principles and ergonomically correct postures and movements.

essential professionalism and image

Why are professionalism and my image so important to my success in cosmetology or a related field?

Professionalism has been defined as the conduct, aims, or qualities that characterize or mark a *professional* person. The cosmetology industry and all related fields such as nail technology, barbering, esthetics, and massage therapy represent the "image" industry. There is no other profession in which image and communication skills (which we will learn more about in Chapter 4) are more essential. As a student in training and as a professional, you will come in contact with numerous clients on a daily basis.

Psychologists tell us that people form an opinion of us in the first few seconds of meeting us. It is up to us to make that first impression a positive one. It is also up to us to make that positive impression a lasting one. We can accomplish that by understanding how to enjoy both personal and professional health. This chapter will help you do just that.

essential
concepts

What are the essentials about image and professional development?

As a professional licensee in the cosmetology industry or related career path, it will be essential for you to concentrate on your personal and professional health. You will need to be aware of your physical presence, your nutrition, and your ability to manage your personal stress. In the process, you will realize the importance of developing a positive, winning attitude and practicing professionalism at all times. Chapter 3 of the textbook and this Essential Companion will provide the road map for helping you achieve all these important personal and professional goals.

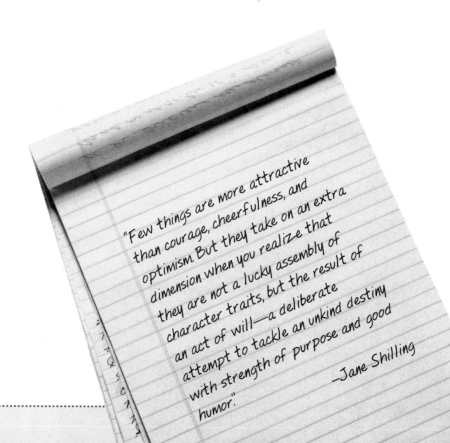

"Few things are more attractive than courage, cheerfulness, and optimism. But they take on an extra dimension when you realize that they are not a lucky assembly of character traits, but the result of an act of will—a deliberate attempt to tackle an unkind destiny with strength of purpose and good humor".

—Jane Shilling

essential ①experience

What Does Your Professional Image Say about You?

Professional image is the impression you project and consists of your outward appearance as well as the conduct you exhibit in the workplace. It is essentially the code of behavior by which you conduct yourself. It relates to proper conduct and business dealings with employers, clients and co-workers, and others with whom you come in contact. Professionalism will help you establish a well-respected reputation. Ask yourself the following questions to help you evaluate your professionalism and your professional image.

1. Do you treat others honestly and fairly at all times?

2. Are you courteous and do you show respect for the feelings, beliefs, and rights of others?

3. Do you keep your word when you make a promise?

4. Do you set an example of good conduct and behavior at all times?

5. Are you loyal to your family, your friends, your school, and fellow students?

6. Do you obey all the rules and standards of conduct set forth by your institution?

If you answered "no" to any of the above questions, you may want to reevaluate your commitment to a professional career. If you answered "yes" to all, give yourself a pat on the back. You practice many qualities required for projecting a professional image.

essential
2 experience

Policy Development

Imagine yourself the owner of a professional establishment and write a detailed dress code that you would require all employees to follow.

DRESS CODE:

_____

_____

_____

_____

_____

_____

_____

_____

_____

_____

_____

_____

_____

_____

_____

_____

_____

essential
experience
3

Word Scramble—Your Professional Image

Scramble	Correct Word
csexeeir	_ _ _ _ _ _ _ _ *Clue:* Promotes proper functions of organs
ggnmoior	_ _ _ _ _ _ _ _ *Clue:* An extension of personal hygiene
loanitaxre	_ _ _ _ _ _ _ _ _ _ *Clue:* Getting away from it all.
oeptrus	_ _ _ _ _ _ _ *Clue:* Position or bearing of the body
rtoutniin	_ _ _ _ _ _ _ _ _ *Clue:* Taking in and utilizing food substances
stre	_ _ _ _ *Clue:* Recovery from fatigue
csimongreo	_ _ _ _ _ _ _ _ _ _ *Clue:* the study of human characteristics for the specific work environment
niosfedorpliamsi	_ _ _ _ _ _ _ _ _ _ _ _ _ _ _ _ *Clue:* business conduct
ehhtal	_ _ _ _ _ _ *Clue:* well-being
neegyih	_ _ _ _ _ _ _ *Clue:* practicing cleanliness
ressst	_ _ _ _ _ _ *Clue:* inability to cope
ardhtyde	_ _ _ _ _ _ _ _ *Clue:* combined with water
ciborea	_ _ _ _ _ _ _ *Clue:* active
hcettrsngi	_ _ _ _ _ _ _ _ *Clue:* enhances flexibility

essential
4 experience

Rate Your Image

On a scale of 1 to 5, with 5 considered the best, rate your appearance in the following categories:

_____ Clothing is clean, pressed, and free of stains or damage.

_____ Dress is in compliance with the dress code established by the institution.

_____ Shoes are clean, polished, and in good repair.

_____ Makeup (if applicable) is tasteful and neatly applied.

_____ Hair is properly groomed and styled appropriately for current trends.

_____ Facial hair (beard or mustache, if applicable) is properly trimmed and neat.

_____ Hands and nails are properly manicured; nails are clean and trimmed appropriately.

_____ Fragrance is appropriate, not overpowering.

_____ Hygiene is maintained (daily bath, proper use of deodorant, teeth are brushed, and so on).

_____ Jewelry is kept to a minimum and not overdone or too trendy.

Add your scores and evaluate your image according to the following guidelines.

45–50	Your image is excellent.
40–44	Your image is above average.
30–39	Your image is average.
Below 30	Improvement is needed. Evaluate the chart and pay particular attention to any category rated less than 3. Make a personal commitment to improvement in those areas.

essential
experience
5

Analyze Your Personal Lifestyle

Answer the following questions thoughtfully and honestly.

1. How many hours of sleep do you get on average nightly?

_____

2. Describe the exercise you get daily/weekly, if any.

_____

_____

3. What methods do you use for relaxation, and how often do you use them?

_____

_____

4. Describe your daily personal hygiene and grooming regimen including the care of your hands and feet.

_____

_____

5. Think back over the past three days and report on your nutrition habits. What did you eat for breakfast, lunch, and dinner over that period of time?

_____

_____

6. Evaluate and list other lifestyle components such as the use of alcohol, tobacco, or drugs. Do they have a negative impact on your life?

_____

_____

As a result of the analysis of your personal lifestyle, write a "Plan of Action" for improving your lifestyle and habits to make the most of a healthy and balanced life, physically, mentally, and emotionally.

Plan of Action

_____

_____

_____

_____

essential
experience
6

Create a Fitness Program

Design a personal fitness regimen based on guidelines found in the chapter. Incorporate the following elements:

- Thirty minutes of exercise daily at least five times per week
- aerobic activity

- stretching activities
- weight-bearing activities

Follow the regimen completely for one full week. At the conclusion of one week, evaluate the effectiveness of the plan by answering the following questions:

1. Did you experience a feeling of personal accomplishment?

_____

2. Did you find that you have muscles you didn't seem to know existed?

_____

3. Did you find the regimen easier to commit to than you thought possible?

_____

4. Did you feel better?

_____

5. Did you experience a higher level of energy?

_____

6. Did you lose any weight or inches?

_____

7. Do the results warrant following the regimen for one more week, then, perhaps, another week?

_____

essential
7 experience

Your Attitude—What Does It Say About You?

One way to determine whether or not you possess and convey a positive attitude is to ask yourself the following questions daily. They have been adapted from a well-known poem, "I Promise Myself," by an unknown author.

1. Do you promise yourself to be so strong that nothing can disturb your peace of mind?

2. Do you promise yourself to talk health, happiness, and prosperity to every person you meet?

3. Do you promise yourself to make all your friends feel that there is something special in them?

4. Do you promise yourself to look at the sunny side of everything and make your optimism come true?

5. Do you promise yourself to think only of the BEST, to work only for the BEST, and to expect only the BEST?

6. Do you promise yourself to be just as enthusiastic about the success of others as you are about your own success?

7. Do you promise yourself to forget the mistakes of the past and press on to the greater achievements of the future?

8. Do you promise yourself to wear a cheerful countenance at all times and greet every living creature you meet with a smile?

9. Do you promise yourself to give so much time to the improvement of yourself that you have no time to criticize others?

10. Do you promise yourself to be too large for worry, too noble for anger, too strong for fear, and too happy to permit the presence of trouble in your life?

If you make these ten promises daily, you will live a life full of prosperity and rewards too great to count!

essential review

Using the following words, fill in the blanks below to form a thorough review of Chapter 3, "Your Professional Image."

aesthetically	flexibility	personal	stability
balance	forty	personality	stress
callused	harmoniously	pressure	tension
cleanse	impression	professional	thirty
dimensional	lower back	self-awareness	varicose veins
disconnect	mind	shock absorption	weight
energy	natural	simple	work habits
ergonomics	osteoporosis	sleep	
fifty	oxygenating	soles	

1. Your professional image is the _____ you project and consists of your outward appearance and the conduct you exhibit in the workplace.

2. Adequate _____ is essential for good health.

3. An adequate fitness program includes exercises to accomplish aerobic strength, _____, and endurance.

4. The daily maintenance of cleanliness and healthfulness is known as _____ hygiene.

5. A professional in cosmetology should practice _____ management through relaxation, rest, and exercise.

6. Physical presentation, which includes your posture, your walk, and your movements, is part of your _____ image.

7. The nutrients in food supply the body with _____ and ensure proper body functions.

8. Good health means the body, _____, and spirit are all working together cooperatively.

9. Eating poorly, smoking, drinking in excess, taking drugs, skipping exercise, holding on to toxic emotions, and lacking a sense of purpose all cause the mind to _____ from the body.

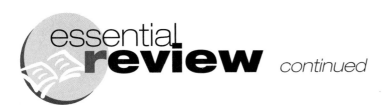

essential **review** *continued*

10. Achieving _____ in your life—between what you want for yourself and what others want for you, between work and play, between self-interest and a sensitivity to others—is the key to leading a happy and productive life.

11. We should _____, moisturize, exfoliate, and protect our bodily and facial skin with a regular skin-care regimen.

12. Many salon owners consider appearance, _____, and poise to be just as important for success as technical knowledge and skills.

13. When you obtain employment, strive to have your hair, makeup, and clothing style blend _____ with your surroundings.

14. Choose clothing that is functional as well as _____ pleasing, but which also falls within the salon's dress code.

15. Accessories are best kept _____ and attractive, whether hair ornamentation, scarves, jewelry, belts, or ties.

16. Using color products such as _____ coloring, blonding, highlights, and gray hair coverage will work as excellent advertisements to help you sell those services to your clients.

17. A clean, _____ approach in makeup is key to presenting yourself professionally.

18. Stress can also be thought of as any situation that causes _____ .

19. Establishing a daily routine of going to bed and getting up at the same time and taking meals at the same time helps promote balance and _____ in life.

20. There are _____ specific nutrients in our food that fall into the categories of carbohydrates, proteins, fats, vitamins, minerals, and water.

21. Maintain a healthy _____ by eating sensible portions, taking meals in a calm environment, and chew each bite of food thoroughly.

22. Water is responsible for a wide variety of metabolic functions including _____ the blood and giving us energy.

23. Use weight-bearing activities to build muscle and develop a leaner, fat-burning body which helps prevent _____.

24. Good posture should be developed early in life and then reinforced through _____ and regular physical activity.

essential review *continued*

25. When giving a manicure or a facial, sit with the _____ against the chair, leaning slightly forward.

26. When giving a manicure, sit with your back straight and keep the entire _____ of your feet on the floor.

27. Scientists have determined that high heels of any style apply _____ to the knees.

28. Low-heeled, wider shoes that spread _____ on the foot and give the toes more room will give you the support and balance to help maintain good posture and offset fatigue.

29. Elevating your feet periodically throughout the day will give the vascular system in the legs a much-needed rest, however brief, and may prevent _____.

30. A pedicure that includes cleansing, removal of _____ skin, massage, and toenail trims will keep your feet at their best.

31. An awareness of your body posture and movements, coupled with better _____ and proper tools and equipment, will greatly enhance your health and comfort.

32. _____ is an applied science concerned with designing and arranging things people use so that the people and things interact most efficiently and safely.

essential
discoveries and accomplishments

In the space below, jot some notes about what concepts of this chapter were hardest for you to understand or remember. Imagine finding yourself suddenly in the role of "teacher" and consider what you would tell your "students" about these difficult concepts.

Share your *Essential Discoveries* with some of the other students in your class and ask if they are helpful to them. You may want to revise your notes based on good ideas shared by your peers. Under "Accomplishments," list at least three things you have accomplished since your last entry that relate to your career goals.

Discoveries:

_____

_____

_____

_____

_____

Accomplishments:

_____

_____

_____

_____

_____

_____

_____

Communicating for Success

essential **objectives**

After studying this chapter and completing the Essential
Companion *components, you should be able to:*

1. Explain the basic processes of effective communication.

2. Assess a client's needs based on the "total look" concept.

3. Conduct a successful client consultation.

4. Handle delicate communication with your clients.

5. Build open lines of communication with coworkers and salon managers.

essential communication skills

Why do I need to learn about communicating when I just want to cut hair?

Today's professionals, regardless of their chosen field, thrive on the exchange of information. In fact, it is information that acts as the fuel that keeps businesses going, moving, and growing. You must think of managing your career as a professional cosmetologist as that of managing your own business. Indeed, when you build and retain a loyal clientele, you are building a successful business. Therefore, you need to receive information in order to make decisions, develop strategies, and effectively interact with your clients. You need to send information if you want your decisions and strategies to be followed and accepted.

This exchange of information is called communication. Your technical skills, however outstanding they may be, will not bring back a client who does not feel comfortable, appreciated, and important as a result of a visit to your salon. Thus, you must be able to address those important social and emotional needs through effective communications. In addition, you cannot provide those exceptional technical services if you do not truly understand the clients' desires. Therefore, communication skills play a huge role in your quest for success.

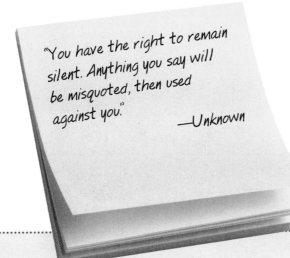

"You have the right to remain silent. Anything you say will be misquoted, then used against you."

—Unknown

essential concepts for communicating effectively

What do I need to know about communicating in order to provide quality service to my clients and enjoy career success?

We communicate not only by speaking but by listening, reading, and writing. In order to exchange information with our clients about their hair, skin, and nail care needs, we must be able to exchange information effectively. We send information by speaking and writing. We receive information by listening and reading. In addition to those methods, we communicate without using words. We can send and receive messages by using gestures, facial expressions, voice changes, eye contact, personal mannerisms, dress, and posture. Throughout this whole communicating process, we are involved in relationship building. We will build relationships with our clients, with our coworkers, and with our supervisors and salon managers or owners.

Therefore, we must develop exceptional skills in conducting consultations with our clients that will result in their desired outcomes. We must learn to interact effectively on a day-to-day basis with our peers and coworkers in order to participate in a highly productive, team-oriented environment. And, finally, we must know how to respond to and interact favorably with our supervisors in order to ensure our continued career development and growth.

essential experience

1

Body Language Matching Exercise

Every part of our body has something to add to the message we are trying to send. Hand movements are the most common companions to spoken messages, more so for some than others. Many hand movements are so common they have come to mean the same thing for all of us. From the list below, match the listed hand movements with the nonverbal message they send.

1. Pointing a finger at someone   ____ Boredom, nervousness

2. Twiddling thumbs   ____ A warning, an accusation

3. Clasping two hands overhead   ____ Hopefulness

4. Drumming or tapping fingers   ____ Calmness, self-confidence

5. Crossing two fingers   ____ A threat

6. Crossing arms across chest   ____ Impatience, annoyance

7. Folding hands together on desk   ____ "Okay" or "right on"

8. Making a circle with one's thumb and forefinger.   ____ Authority, anger

9. Making a fist   ____ Victory

essential
2 experience

Eye Movement

As with our hands, we can use our eyes to send nonverbal messages which might include close attention, anger, admiration, disbelief, or surprise. Study the list of various eye movements below and write in the space provided the nonverbal message you believe the eye movement sends.

Staring and having a tightened jaw   _____

Rolling the eyes   _____

Looking directly at someone   _____

Opening the eyes wide   _____

Staring/glaring at someone for too long   _____

Blinking eyes rapidly   _____

Looking directly at strangers in close quarters   _____

Shifting eyes away to avoid direct contact   _____

essential experience

3

Mind Map Consultation Interference

Mind mapping simply creates a free-flowing outline of material or information with the central or key point being located in the center. The key point of this mind map is a client consultation. Diagram all the things that could interfere with the communication process during a client consultation. Use words, pictures, and symbols as desired. Use color to increase the mind's retention and memory of the material. Keep your mind open and uncluttered and don't worry about where a line or word should go, as the organization of the map will usually take care of itself.

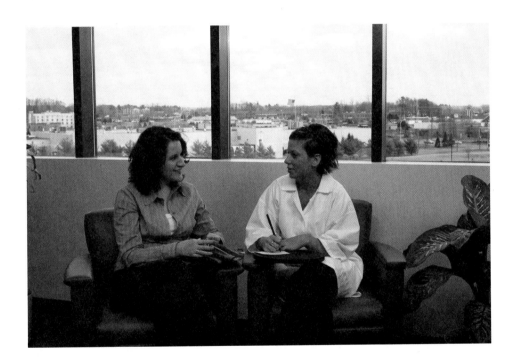

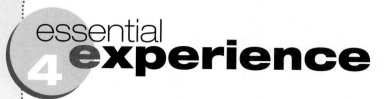

essential
4 experience

Partner Messaging

Choose another student as your partner and conduct this communication exercise. Spend five minutes talking to each other about any subject you choose. Interact openly and respond to each other naturally. At the conclusion of the five minutes, each of you should make a list of the messages you received. Then review the lists together and compare the messages received to the messages you each intended to send. List the results in the space provided.

Message Received	Message Intended
_____	_____
_____	_____
_____	_____
_____	_____
_____	_____
_____	_____
_____	_____
_____	_____
_____	_____

essential experience

5

Role-Playing a Dissatisfied Client

The purpose of role-playing is to help you understand the views and feelings of other people with respect to a wide range of personal and social issues. By acting out situations in which people are in conflict, you can begin to understand the other person's point of view. In this activity there will be three main characters, and several other students will be needed to observe. Three of you will perform the role-playing exercise while the other students observe and make notes. Upon completion of the role-play, ask the observers what they saw, what worked in the communication exchange, what did not work, and why.

One student will role-play the salon stylist, another student will play a client who has come into the salon for a haircolor service and is clearly dissatisfied with the results. The third character will be the salon supervisor who ultimately has to become involved in the quest for a solution. Upon completion of the role-play and discussion with the observers, record your findings from the activity in the space provided. Consider answering the following questions: What did you learn from this experience? Are there certain ways to handle conflict that are more effective than others? If so, what are they and why do they work better?

_____

_____

_____

_____

_____

_____

_____

_____

essential experience

6

Windowpane—Client Consultation Tools

Windowpaning is the process of transferring key elements, points, or steps in a lesson into visual images that are hand sketched into the squares or "panes" of a matrix. Let your mind think in pictures and sketch the essential concepts printed in each of the following windowpanes. Don't be concerned with your artistic ability. Use lines and stick figures to depict the concepts requested.

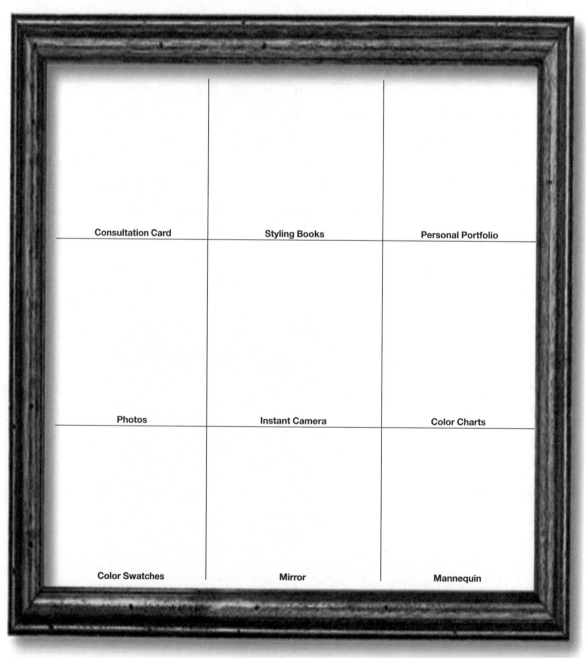

Consultation Card	Styling Books	Personal Portfolio
Photos	Instant Camera	Color Charts
Color Swatches	Mirror	Mannequin

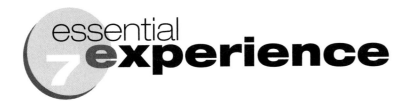

essential
experience
7

Topics to Avoid

In the space provided make a list of at least six topics that you should avoid discussing with clients. Then write a brief explanation as to why these topics would be inappropriate, and list alternative topics that you might suggest if the client should bring up any of the inappropriate ones.

Explanation and Alternative Topics:

_____

_____

_____

_____

_____

_____

_____

_____

_____

_____

_____

_____

_____

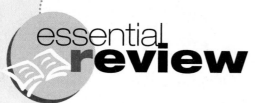

essential **review**

True or False

Circle T for True or F for False as applicable to the following statements.

T F 1. Your ability to form satisfying relationships with your clients is a key factor in determining if cosmetology will be just a job for you or a fulfilling career.

T F 2. Communication is the act or instance of transmitting information, in the form of symbols, gestures, or behaviors, in order to express an idea or concept so that it is barely understood.

T F 3. The first step in the communication process is to collect your thoughts and feelings of what you want others to understand.

T F 4. The second step in the communication process is to translate your thoughts and feelings into symbols that can be easily understood by others.

T F 5. You may need to help your clients articulate, or vaguely express, their true wants and desires by providing them with symbols they can adopt as their own.

T F 6. Clutter is any type of distraction that can keep you from focusing on the conversation you are having with your client.

T F 7. Reflective listening is the process of repeating back to the client, in your own words, what you think he or she is telling you.

T F 8. If a client doesn't fully realize that his or her choice in a service will not benefit him or her, it is your obligation to find a way to bluntly let the client know.

T F 9. The final step in interpreting the client's message consists of misunderstanding all the clues and symbols the client is putting out.

T F 10. The verbal communication with a client that is used to determine the client's desired results is called a client consultation.

T F 11. The client consultation creates the opportunity to direct his or her attention to other clients visiting the salon.

T F 12. Hair swatches are very durable because they are generally made from real hair fibers.

T   F   **13.** A consultation prior to a nail service is best done at the manicure table, as long as it is a comfortable place to talk.

T   F   **14.** A skin care consultation should take place in the reception area so you can speak candidly about the client's skin care issues.

T   F   **15.** A consultation with a first-time client should be scheduled at least ten minutes prior to the actual appointment.

T   F   **16.** Handing a new client a style book or magazine that is torn or is missing pages looks tacky and amateurish.

T   F   **17.** If the client is having a hard time explaining the look he or she desires, clarify the meaning by asking short and direct questions.

T   F   **18.** Record any formulations or products used, including the strength and any specific techniques followed, on the Rolodex.

T   F   **19.** To earn a client's trust and loyalty, always approach a new client with a smile on your face.

T   F   **20.** When meeting a client for the first time, always introduce yourself.

T   F   **21.** Don't try to fake your clients into thinking you are someone or something that you are not.

T   F   **22.** If a client arrives late, you should establish a precedent by refusing to complete the service under any circumstances.

T   F   **23.** If a client shows up at an incorrect time or day, politely explain the mistake and offer to reschedule.

T   F   **24.** Never argue with a client or try to force your opinion on him or her.

T   F   **25.** Using unkind words or actions with regard to your colleagues is sometimes necessary.

essential
discoveries and
accomplishments

In the space below, jot some notes about what concepts of this chapter were hardest for you to understand or remember. Imagine finding yourself suddenly in the role of "teacher" and consider what you would tell your "students" about these difficult concepts.

Share your *Essential Discoveries* with some of the other students in your class and ask if they are helpful to them. You may want to revise your notes based on good ideas shared by your peers. Under "Accomplishments," list at least three things you have accomplished since your last entry that relate to your career goals.

Discoveries:

_____

_____

_____

_____

_____

Accomplishments:

_____

_____

_____

_____

_____

_____

Infection Control: Principles and Practice

essential objectives

After studying this chapter and completing the Essential Companion *components, you should be able to:*

1. List the types and classifications of bacteria.

2. Describe how bacteria grow and reproduce.

3. Explain the difference between bacteria and viruses.

4. Describe vegetable and animal parasites that may be seen in the salon.

5. Define AIDS and hepatitis and explain how they are transmitted.

6. Explain the differences between sterilization, disinfection, and sanitation.

7. Discuss how to safely handle and use disinfectant products.

8. Describe how to sanitize and disinfect various salon tools and surfaces.

9. Explain the purpose and use of an MSDS sheet.

10. Discuss universal precautions and your responsibilities as a salon professional.

essential principles and practices of infection control

Why do I need to know about the principles of infection control?

If you work in cosmetology or a related career field, you will come in contact with the public on a regular basis in a variety of ways. Understanding bacteriology, sterilization, and sanitation will make a big difference in how you protect yourself and your clients from the spread of infection or disease. There has never been a time in our history when the public has been more aware of how easily disease can be spread. Your clients' perceptions of you will be greatly improved if you convey both knowledge and concern about bacteria and the spread of disease.

There is an old saying that you never get a second chance to make a positive first impression. Nothing could be more appropriate regarding the first impressions you and your establishment make on the public. They will judge you by the cleanliness of the establishment where you work, by the cleanliness of your work station and implements, and by the neat, well-groomed image you present. Today's public demands that their doctors, their dentists, their optometrists, and their beauty service professionals practice the highest levels of infection control and decontamination. So, if you want to build a solid, repeat clientele for the services in which you specialize, you will want to practice obvious sanitation and disinfection measures to build client confidence and trust in you. In addition, you must be able to take the necessary steps to protect yourself from infection by treating a client who may have an infectious disease you can't identify.

"Pessimism becomes a self-fulfilling prophecy. The good news is — optimism does too. Since you're free to choose, choose success and happiness. Choose optimism."

—Unknown

essential concepts

What are the essential concepts of providing the safest possible environment using effective decontamination and infection control procedures?

As a professional in the cosmetology industry, you will need to understand the difference between nonpathogenic (helpful or harmless) and pathogenic (harmful) bacteria. You will need to know the various classifications of bacteria and how to identify each. It is essential that you develop an understanding of bacterial growth and reproduction, bacterial infections, other infectious agents, immunity, and acquired immune deficiency syndrome (AIDS).

As a successful licensee in the field of cosmetology or related discipline, you will need to know about both prevention and control. You need to understand that surfaces may be contaminated even if they appear clean; you will also need to know the steps necessary to make those surfaces germ free. You will learn about procedures and products for sanitation and sterilization as well as disinfection, and will gain knowledge about the tools and implements used to accomplish these tasks. The Occupational Safety and Health Administration (OSHA) plays an important role in the responsibilities of each licensed establishment to ensure a safe work environment both for workers and the public. By taking the approach known as universal precautions and following the same infection control practices with all clients, regardless of their health status, you are ensuring the best possible protection for you and the public.

essential
experience
1

Window Pane

Windowpaning is the process of transferring key elements, points, or steps in a lesson into visual images that are hand sketched into the squares or "panes" of a matrix. Let your mind think in pictures and sketch the essential concepts printed in each of the following windowpanes.

Bacteria Window Pane

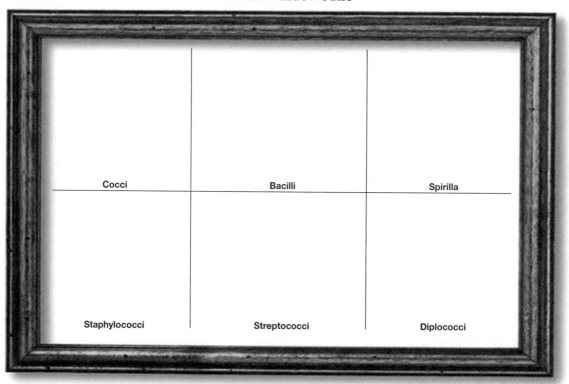

Cocci	Bacilli	Spirilla
Staphylococci	Streptococci	Diplococci

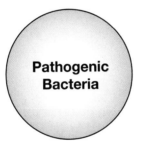

essential
experience
2

Mind Map

Mind mapping creates a free-flowing outline of material or information. Using the central or key point of Pathogenic Bacteria, diagram the different classifications and characteristics of harmful bacteria, the conditions they cause, and the areas where they may be found. Use words, pictures, and symbols as desired. Using color will increase your memory of the material.

Pathogenic Bacteria

essential
3 experience

Matching Terms

Match the following essential terms with their identifying terms or phrases.

Activity A

_____ Bacilli

_____ Bacteriology

_____ Contagious

_____ Diplococci

_____ Fungi

_____ Local infection

_____ Motility

_____ Nonpathogenic

_____ Pediculosis

_____ Scabies

_____ Staphylococci

1. Self-movement

2. Grow in bunches

3. Causes pneumonia

4. Mold, mildew, yeasts

5. Boil, pimple

6. Itch mite

7. Lice

8. Helpful/harmless bacteria

9. Communicable

10. Study of microorganisms

11. Cause influenza and typhoid fever

Activity B

_____ Bacteria

_____ Cocci

_____ Flagella

_____ Microbes

_____ Pathogenic

_____ Protoplasm

_____ Spirilla

_____ Streptococci

1. Harmful bacteria

2. Minute, one-celled, vegetable microorganisms

3. Grow in chains

4. Round-shaped organisms

5. Hair-like projections

6. Corkscrew-shaped organisms

7. Material needed to sustain life

8. Germs

essential
4 experience

Client Protection

Imagine that you own a professional establishment. You are committed to maintaining the highest levels of sanitation and client protection possible. Take a tour through your establishment and identify and list the areas in the salon that are most susceptible to pathogenic bacteria.

_____

_____

_____

_____

_____

_____

_____

_____

_____

_____

_____

_____

_____

essential
5 experience

Word Scramble—Bacteriology

Scramble	Correct Word
aasseptir	_ _ _ _ _ _ _ _ _
	Clue: Require living matter for growth
abemlcicnoum	_ _ _ _ _ _ _ _ _ _ _
	Clue: Contagious
aiarcetb	_ _ _ _ _ _ _ _
	Clue: Minute, one-celled vegetable microorganisms
aiibllc	_ _ _ _ _ _ _
	Clue: Short, rod-shaped organisms
alcicyoocshpt	_ _ _ _ _ _ _ _ _ _ _ _ _
	Clue: Grow in bunches or clusters
asseibc	_ _ _ _ _ _ _
	Clue: Caused by an itch mite
calii	_ _ _ _ _
	Clue: Its whip-like motion propels bacteria in liquid
cesmpoorci	_ _ _ _ _ _ _ _ _ _
	Clue: Viewing instrument
cpnaiegoht	_ _ _ _ _ _ _ _ _ _
	Clue: Disease producing
leaglafl	_ _ _ _ _ _ _ _
	Clue: Hairlike projections
iisyhlps	_ _ _ _ _ _ _ _
	Clue: Sexually transmitted disease
ilotymit	_ _ _ _ _ _ _ _
	Clue: Self-movement
maosloptrp	_ _ _ _ _ _ _ _ _ _
	Clue: Colorless, jellylike substance

essential
experience *continued*
5

Word Scramble—Bacteriology

Scramble	Correct Word
mrseg	_ _ _ _ _ _
	Clue: Also known as bacteria
napnocnghieot	_ _ _ _ _ _ _ _ _ _ _ _ _
	Clue: Helpful or harmless
calol fctnmoiine	_ _ _ _ _ _ _ _ _ _ _ _ _
	Clue: Contains pus
orsiocpcctet	_ _ _ _ _ _ _ _ _ _ _ _
	Clue: Cause infections such as strep throat
seborcim	_ _ _ _ _ _ _ _ _
	Clue: Also known as germs or bacteria
ssriminagoorcm	_ _ _ _ _ _ _ _ _ _ _ _ _ _
	Clue: Bacteria are an example of this
staoeyhprps	_ _ _ _ _ _ _ _ _ _ _
	Clue: Live on dead matter, not disease producing
ucosaignto	_ _ _ _ _ _ _ _ _ _
	Clue: Spreads by contact
uicedsslpoi	_ _ _ _ _ _ _ _ _ _ _
	Clue: Head lice

essential
experience
6

Jeopardy

As in the game *Jeopardy,* write questions that would be correctly answered as follows:

Bacteriology for $100

1. The science that deals with the study of microorganisms called bacteria.

_____

2. Minute, one-celled vegetable microorganisms found nearly everywhere.

_____

3. Also known as germs or microbes, they can exist almost anywhere on the skin of the body or in water, air, decayed matter, secretions of body openings, on clothing, and beneath the nails.

_____

Bacteriology for $200

1. Organisms which perform many useful functions such as decomposing refuse and improving soil fertility.

_____

2. Nonpathogenic bacteria which live on dead matter and do not produce disease.

_____

3. Disease producing when they invade plant or animal tissue.

_____

Bacteriology for $300

1. The colorless, jellylike substance in which food elements such as proteins, fats, carbohydrates, mineral salts, and water are present.

_____

2. The stage in which microorganisms grow and reproduce.

_____

essential experience *continued*

6

Bacteriology for $400

1. Living organisms that are so small they can pass through the pores of a porcelain filter.

_____

2. Molds, mildews, and yeasts which can produce contagious diseases such as ringworm and favus.

_____

3. These are responsible for contagious diseases and conditions, such as head lice.

_____

Bacteriology for $500

1. The ability of the body to destroy bacteria that have gained entrance, and thus resist infection.

_____

2. Something the body develops after it has overcome a disease, or through inoculation.

_____

3. A person who is personally immune to a disease yet can transmit germs to other people.

_____

4. A person can be infected with this for up to eleven years without having symptoms.

_____

5. This is transmitted through unprotected sexual contact, IV drug users sharing needles, and accidents with needles in health care settings.

_____

6. It causes AIDS.

_____

essential
experience
7

Safety and Health Inspection

Complete the following partial Safety and Health Inspection Report, which is adapted from *Safety and Health in the Salon,* for your institution. Write in brief explanations if an area is out of compliance.

Location: _____ Inspected by: _____ Date: _____

All Areas—Housekeeping and Sanitation

Yes　No　There is evidence the facility has been used for cooking or living quarters.

Yes　No　All areas are orderly, dusted, clean, sanitary, well-lighted, and rodent free.

Yes　No　Floors are swept clean and hair is swept up after each client service.

Yes　No　Windows, screens, and curtains are cleaned regularly.

Yes　No　Waste materials are deposited in a metal waste receptacle with a self-closing lid.

Yes　No　Waste receptacles are emptied regularly throughout the day.

Yes　No　All sinks and drinking fountains are cleaned regularly.

Yes　No　Separate or disposable drinking cups are provided for clients, employees, and students.

Yes　No　Hot and cold water faucets are clean and leak-free.

Yes　No　Toilets and washing facilities are clean and sanitary.

Yes　No　Toilet tissue, paper towels, and pump-like antiseptic liquid soap are provided.

Yes　No　Door handles are cleaned regularly.

Yes　No　Food is stored separately from clinic products.

Yes　No　Eating and drinking is done on sanitary surfaces separate from chemical handling or where services are being performed.

Yes　No　Work area is appropriately ventilated for services provided and fans, humidifiers, and exhaust and ventilation systems are regularly cleaned.

Yes　No　Floors are free of water or other substances that could cause a slip, trip, or fall.

Yes　No　MSDS are available for all chemicals used in the clinic.

Yes　No　All chemicals are properly stored and all containers are properly labeled.

essential
experience *continued*
7

Yes	No	Appropriate personal protective equipment (eye protection, gloves, dust and organic vapor masks, and so on) are available and used according to manufacturer's directions and salon policy.
Yes	No	Washing machine provides water temperature of at least 160 degrees Fahrenheit.
Yes	No	Hospital-grade tuberculocidal disinfecting solution and instructions are available for cleaning combs, brushes, plastic capes, and other materials as required.

Emergency Precautions and First Aid

Yes	No	Emergency phone numbers are posted where they can be readily found in an emergency.
Yes	No	Fire evacuation procedures are posted.
Yes	No	First aid kits are readily accessible with necessary supplies.
Yes	No	First aid kit is periodically inspected and replenished as needed.
Yes	No	Emergency eye wash bottles are provided where chemical handling is done and where chemical services are provided.
Yes	No	There is ready access to a sink with tempered water to completely flush the eyes from hazardous materials.
Yes	No	Exit and warning signs (biohazard, fire door, flammable or toxic chemicals) are posted where appropriate.

_____

_____

_____

_____

essential experience

8

Word Search—Decontamination

Word	Clue
_____	There are three widely used forms
_____	This can kill bacteria but is not a disinfectant
_____	Bloodborne pathogens
_____	Causes contamination
_____	Surfaces which look clean may still be this
_____	There are three levels of this
_____	Kills microbes on nonporous surfaces
_____	Controls microorganisms on nonporous surfaces
_____	A gas released from formalin tablets
_____	Sodium Hypochlorite
_____	Provides pertinent information about ingredients
_____	This is part of the United States Department of Labor
_____	Hospital disinfectants must be this
_____	Safe and fast-acting disinfectant
_____	Lowest level of decontamination
_____	Most effective decontamination

After finding the appropriate word from the above clues, locate the word in the following
word search puzzle.

```
A  H  N  O  I  T  C  E  F  N  I  S  I  D  N  S  G
C  L  O  S  A  N  I  T  A  T  I  O  N  O  F  T  C
O  T  C  U  F  Q  P  U  H  G  Z  A  I  S  O  E  S
N  N  E  O  S  X  P  E  G  L  H  T  T  W  R  R  T
T  A  Q  F  H  E  F  Y  M  S  A  A  N  K  M  I  N
A  N  V  A  Q  O  H  B  O  N  U  U  U  X  A  L  A
M  I  M  D  V  Z  L  O  I  Q  V  N  I  W  L  I  T
I  M  H  E  T  O  B  M  L  I  M  T  C  M  D  Z  C
N  A  V  C  M  R  A  F  M  D  K  R  F  N  E  A  E
A  T  L  P  N  T  O  G  D  S  B  Q  C  K  H  T  F
T  N  O  U  N  R  I  C  W  K  D  L  H  C  Y  I  N
E  O  W  O  M  U  J  E  C  C  H  S  E  Z  D  O  I
D  C  C  A  B  R  B  T  S  L  L  P  K  A  E  N  S
T  E  L  S  C  I  T  P  E  S  I  T  N  A  C  E  I
D  I  G  C  I  T  A  M  O  T  P  M  Y  S  A  H  D
N  Z  P  E  M  A  L  Q  O  T  U  A  M  A  E  Y  S
F  I  L  A  D  I  C  A  N  O  M  O  D  U  E  S  P
```

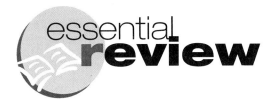

Using the following words, fill in the blanks below to form a thorough review of Chapter 5, "Infection Control: Principles and Practice."

abscesses	diphtheria	natural	ringworm
acquired immunity	disinfectant	nonpathogenic	round-shaped
bacilli	eleven	one-celled	spherical spores
boils	general	outer covering	streptococci
cilia	Hepatitis B	parasites	syphilis
contagious	immunity	pathogenic	twelve
daughter cells	local	pneumonia	virus
decomposing	microscope	protoplasm	viruses
garbage	mitosis	pustules	

1. Staphylococci are pus-forming organisms that grow in clusters and cause

   _____ , _____ , and _____ .

2. Cocci are _____ bacteria that appear singly or in groups.

3. A _____ infection is indicated by a boil or pimple and contains pus.

4. Organisms that live on other living organisms and do not give anything in return are

   known as _____ .

5. The body's ability to destroy bacteria that have gained entrance is called

   _____ .

6. Typhoid fever, tuberculosis, and _____ are examples of bacilli.

7. Two useful functions of nonpathogenic bacteria are improving soil fertility and

   _____ .

8. Bacteria are _____ vegetable microorganisms found nearly everywhere.

9. The most common bacteria, which produce diseases such as tetanus, influenza, typhoid

   fever, and diphtheria, is called _____ .

10. Flagella, a hairlike projection, is also known as _____ .

11. Bacteria consist of an outer cell wall and internal _____ .

12. Contagious diseases and conditions such as _____ should never be treated

   in a school or salon, but referred to a physician.

essential review

13. _____ are living organisms so small that they can pass through the pores of a porcelain filter.

14. The body develops _____ after it has overcome a disease or through inoculation.

15. A person can be infected with HIV-1 for _____ years without having symptoms.

16. Diplococci grow in pairs and cause _____.

17. Saprophytes are _____ bacteria which live on dead matter.

18. Bacteria can be seen only with the aid of a _____.

19. _____ organisms are harmful and produce disease.

20. A _____ infection results when the bloodstream carries the bacteria or virus and its toxins to all parts of the body.

21. When bacteria grow and reach their largest size, they divide and split into two new cells. The division is called _____ and the new cells formed are called _____.

22. Immunity against disease can be _____ or acquired.

23. When a disease becomes _____ it spreads from one person to another.

24. Treponema pallida causes _____.

25. _____ are pus-forming organisms that cause infections such as strep throat.

For the remainder of the review, circle the correct answer to each question.

26. Any surface that is not free of dirt, hair, or microbes is:
    a) sterilized   b) contaminated
    c) sterile   d) disinfected

27. A comb with hair in it or a towel with makeup on it is considered to be:
    a) sterilized   b) contaminated
    c) sterile   d) sanitary

28. The three levels of decontamination are sterilization, disinfection, and:
    a) washing   b) dusting
    c) sweeping   d) sanitation

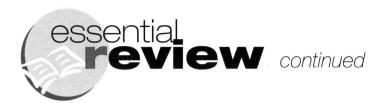

29. The methods of physical sterilization include dry heat and _____.

a) steam autoclave   b) gaseous formaldehyde

c) liquid antiseptic   d) dry sanitation

30. Substances that kill microbes on contaminated tools and other nonporous surfaces are:

a) antiseptics   b) tablets

c) disinfectants   d) liquids

31. Disinfectants must be approved by the:

a) DOE   b) EPA

c) APE   d) DOL

32. Federal law requires manufacturers to provide product information on the:

a) MSDS   b) MDSD

c) SMDS   d) MSSD

33. The Occupational Safety and Health Administration was created as part of the:

a) DOJ   b) DOE

c) DOL   d) DOA

34. Most QUATS disinfect implements within _____ minutes.

a) 5 to 10   b) 10 to 15

c) 15 to 20   d) 20 - 25

35. If salon implements come into contact with blood, they should be cleaned and immersed in:

a) Quaternary Ammonium Compounds   b) Phenolic disinfectants

c) Sodium hypochlorite   d) EPA Registered Disinfectant

36. A disinfectant that was used in the past as an enclosed dry cabinet sanitizer and which is no longer considered safe is:

a) QUATS   b) alcohol

c) bleach   d) formalin

37. The third and lowest level of decontamination is known as:

a) disinfection   b) sterilization

c) sanitation   d) immunization

38. A sanitizer that is not adequate for instruments and surfaces, but is safe for application to the skin, is:

a) antiseptic
b) phenol
c) chloride
d) bleach

39. The technical term for bleach is:

a) sodium chloride
b) sodium hypochlorite
c) sodium clorox
d) sodium hydroxide

40. About half the people who are infected with the Hepatitis B virus or other bloodborne pathogens are:

a) asymptomatic
b) healthy
c) contaminated
d) immune

essential discoveries and accomplishments

In the space below, jot some notes about what concepts of this chapter were hardest for you to understand or remember. Imagine finding yourself suddenly in the role of "teacher" and consider what you would tell your "students" about these difficult concepts.

Share your *Essential Discoveries* with some of the other students in your class and ask if they are helpful to them. You may want to revise your notes based on good ideas shared by your peers. Under "Accomplishments," list at least three things you have accomplished since your last entry that relate to your career goals.

Discoveries:

_____

_____

_____

_____

_____

Accomplishments:

_____

_____

_____

_____

_____

_____

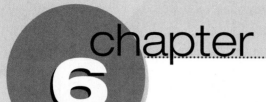

chapter

6

Anatomy and Physiology

essential objectives

After studying this chapter and completing the Essential Companion *components, you should be able to:*

1. Explain the importance of anatomy and physiology to the cosmetology profession.

2. Describe cells, their structure, and their reproduction.

3. Define *tissue* and identify the types of tissues found in the body.

4. Name the ten body systems and explain their basic functions.

5. Demonstrate an understanding of the systems and organs of the human body and their functions.

essential anatomy and physiology

Why do I need to know about cells and the anatomy and physiology of the body when I just want to do hair?

As you do hair and perform all the other services you are qualified and trained to perform, almost without exception you will be affecting the bones, muscles, and nerves of the body. Therefore, it is essential that you understand the basic anatomy and physiology of the body to perform all those services safely and effectively. If you will think about it, you will realize that when you cut hair, you must understand the contours of the head and its bone structure. When you apply makeup, you must perform contouring based on the bone and muscle structure of the face. When giving a scalp treatment, you need to know about the circulatory system in order to achieve maximum stimulation of the scalp, and so forth.

Even though you may not consider studying about anatomy and physiology the most exciting or glamorous part of your training, it is clearly an integral part of your training and will contribute significantly to your effectiveness and success. Certainly your knowledge in this key area will gain your client's trust and establish confidence in your credibility.

essential concepts of anatomy and physiology

What do I need to learn about cells, anatomy, and physiology to be more effective as a cosmetologist?

The cell is the basic structure from which all other body structures are made. You will want to develop a comfortable knowledge about cell growth and metabolism. You will want a basic knowledge of each of the main organs and systems of the body. Once you've gained information about how each organ or system functions and its purpose, you can be more effective in the services you provide.

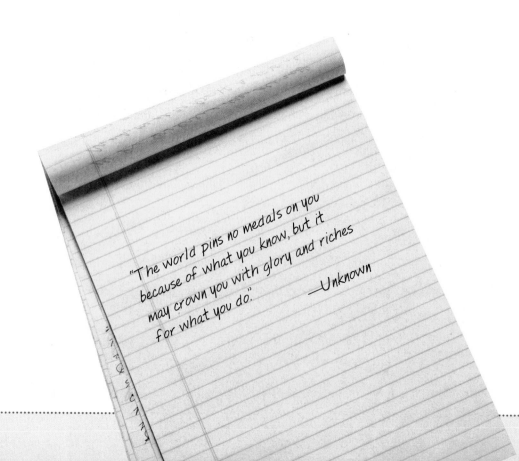

"The world pins no medals on you because of what you know, but it may crown you with glory and riches for what you do."

—Unknown

essential
experience
1

Mind Map—Cell Development

Mind mapping creates a free-flowing outline of material or information. The central or key point is located in the center. The key point of this mind map is the process of development from a basic cell to the various types of tissue to forming organs and developing systems. Using color will increase the mind's retention of the material. Keep your mind open and uncluttered and don't worry about where a line or word should go; the organization of the map will usually take care of itself.

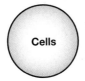

Cells

essential
2 experience

Organs

Label each of the organs indicated in the diagram of a human body. State the purpose of each part of the body in the space provided. You may need to refer to your school's reference library for assistance.

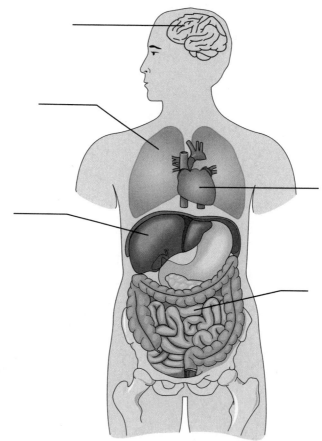

Brain: _____

_____

Heart: _____

_____

Lungs: _____

_____

Liver: _____

_____

Large intestine: _____

_____

essential
③experience

Matching Exercise—Body Systems

Match each of the following essential terms with its definition.

_____ Circulatory

_____ Digestive

_____ Endocrine

_____ Excretory

_____ Integumentary

_____ Muscular

_____ Nervous

_____ Reproductive

_____ Respiratory

_____ Skeletal

1. Duct glands and ductless glands

2. Responsible for changing food into nutrients and waste

3. The physical foundation or framework of the body

4. Situated in the chest cavity, protected by the ribs

5. Covers, shapes, and supports the skeleton; produces all body movements

6. Made up of the skin and its various accessory organs

7. Organs for producing offspring

8. Controls and coordinates the functions of all the other systems and makes them work harmoniously and efficiently

9. Kidneys, liver, skin, intestines and lungs; purifies the body by eliminating waste matter

10. Controls the steady circulation of the blood

essential
4 experience

Word Search—The Muscular System

After identifying the correct word from the clues provided, locate the words in the word search puzzle.

Word	Clue
_____	Separates the fingers
_____	The middle part of the muscle
_____	The muscle between the upper and lower jaws
_____	Draws the eyebrow down and in
_____	Large, thick, triangular-shaped muscle, covers the shoulder
_____	A broad muscle that covers the top of the skull
_____	Bends the wrist, draws the hand up, and closes the fingers toward the forearm
_____	The chewing muscle
_____	Situated at the tip of the chin
_____	The study of the structure, functions, and disease of the muscles

```
C  Z  R  A  Z  S  I  L  A  T  N  E  M  B  D  L
W  Y  D  X  K  J  T  H  K  Q  C  Y  U  E  F  V
N  Z  L  T  Q  X  T  S  J  H  T  C  L  I  A  L
U  J  M  L  L  D  V  H  E  M  C  T  M  G  B  Z
S  U  C  V  E  T  K  S  H  I  O  B  H  B  T  U
P  D  W  M  L  B  F  E  N  I  M  L  S  M  H  U
R  D  X  O  F  U  R  A  D  Z  W  P  U  K  T  E
E  U  Z  C  V  W  T  O  A  S  E  W  Q  P  F  V
T  Q  H  U  D  O  M  N  T  B  R  X  J  M  I  Z
E  Z  D  C  R  Y  B  B  W  A  D  O  Q  A  K  P
S  I  Q  X  O  Z  Q  B  I  G  G  U  X  Y  S  S
S  O  V  L  D  H  O  Z  R  Q  C  U  C  E  G  M
A  Z  O  G  Q  L  E  E  J  W  I  Z  R  T  L  B
M  G  O  O  U  K  Y  U  Y  C  Z  O  G  R  O  F
Y  O  G  T  P  X  N  K  J  H  A  R  U  L  O  R
E  P  I  C  R  A  N  I  U  S  E  L  R  E  B  C
```

essential
5 experience

Word Search—The Muscular System

After identifying the correct word from the clues provided, locate the words in the word search puzzle.

Word	Clue
_____	Forms a flat band around the upper and lower lips
_____	The part of the muscle that does not move
_____	A broad muscle that extends from the chest and shoulder muscles to the side of the chin
_____	Covers the bridge of the nose
_____	Found in the forearm and turns the hand inward
_____	Extends from the masseter muscle to the angle of the mouth
_____	Striped or voluntary muscular tissue
_____	Rotates the shoulder blade and controls the swinging movement of the arm
_____	Large muscle that covers the entire back of the upper arm

```
T  O  P  R  O  C  E  R  U  S  O  F  U  Q  R  A
B  R  R  S  T  R  I  A  T  E  D  R  C  W  I  L
X  R  A  B  Y  A  Q  N  K  H  A  G  W  M  I  B
U  I  C  P  I  A  S  C  C  T  J  H  P  K  X  S
B  S  Y  S  E  C  Q  Z  J  S  N  K  S  I  R  Y
F  O  B  I  C  Z  U  Q  N  I  I  B  Q  O  G  R
J  R  J  Q  J  N  I  L  S  Y  U  D  T  H  M  T
E  I  X  V  H  V  L  U  A  E  V  A  J  A  R  H
A  U  N  V  U  R  K  R  S  R  N  K  V  E  H  R
M  S  N  J  F  G  V  I  T  O  I  G  Y  Q  C  H
S  H  A  M  V  S  N  R  R  J  N  S  B  Q  V  G
Y  P  I  M  M  R  I  P  H  I  G  I  O  Q  E  Y
T  K  N  F  J  C  V  A  E  D  A  X  G  R  Q  Y
A  Z  U  Q  E  Z  A  A  M  X  M  H  D  I  I  I
L  R  L  P  G  H  I  C  V  K  G  S  J  P  R  S
P  R  S  F  L  E  A  I  Z  L  N  S  O  D  L  O
```

essential
experience
6

Crossword Puzzle

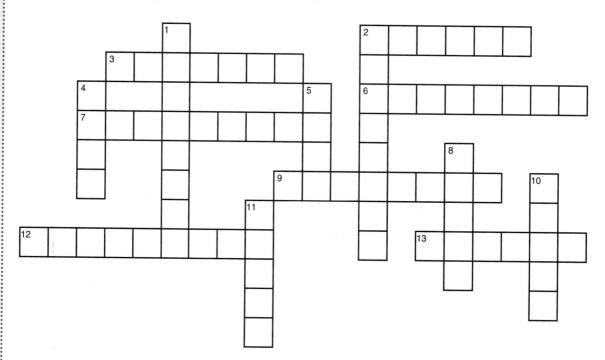

Across

2. Chest
3. Oval, bony case that shapes the top of the head
6. Lower jawbone—strongest bone of the face
7. Forms the lower back part of the cranium
9. Small fragile bones located at the front of the inner wall of the eye socket
12. Scientific study of bones, their structure and functions
13. Wrist

Down

1. Forms the sides and top of the cranium
2. Forms the sides of the head in the ear region
4. Hardest tissue of the body
5. Large bone on the little finger side of the forearm
8. Forms the bridge of the nose
10. Skeleton of the head
11. Adam's apple

essential 7 experience

Bones and Muscles of the Cranium

Using an old shaved mannequin or a Styrofoam head block, draw a line from the center front "hairline" to the center nape. On side one, draw in and label the bones of the head. On side two, draw in and label the muscles of the head. In the absence of a shaved mannequin or Styrofoam head block, you can use the diagrams on this page.

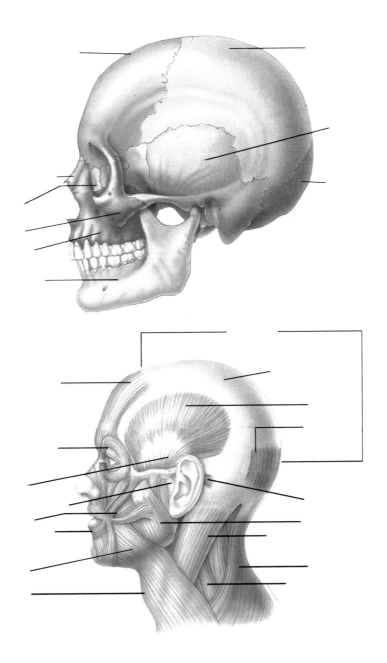

essential
experience
8

Cranial Nerves

On the diagram, label each of the nerves in the head, face, and neck and indicate which are the 5th, 7th, or 11th cranial nerves. Using the number assigned to each nerve, state the area affected by the nerve in the space provided below.

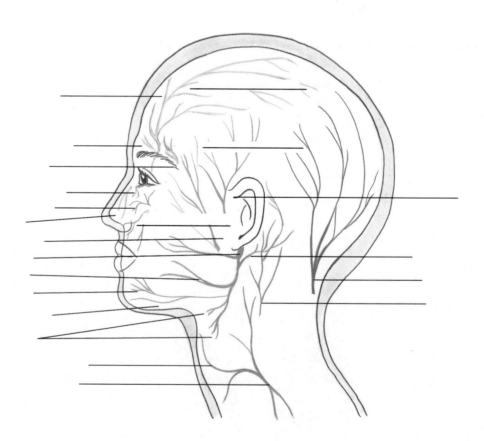

essential experience

Word Search—Circulatory System

After determining the correct words from the clues provided, locate the words in the word search puzzle.

Word	Clue
_____	Artery that supplies the side of the nose
_____	Thick-walled muscular and elastic tubes that carry pure blood from the heart to the capillaries
_____	Upper right or left, thin-walled chambers of the heart
_____	The nutritive fluid circulating through the circulatory system
_____	Minute, thin-walled blood vessels that connect smaller arteries to veins
_____	The main source of blood supply to the head, face, and neck
_____	The artery that supplies the forehead
_____	Internal and external; veins through which blood returns to the heart from the head, face, and neck
_____	White corpuscles

```
Y R L D R L A W X C K T C W S M
R C A Z I Y Q Y D E F Z L E U L
E U A L I T Y K I R D S I I J V
T A S O U A O Y F R I R R E C A
Q A D N I G M R G Z A T H N A R
Y I B S Y L U G A L A C D I R B
S Y E E B I J J L C L J R G P N
E Z I C Y D C I A A N M L S E A
T F K K Z J P R Y G N O D B P F
Y D R E Q A T L J T H G M R Z E
C H N Z C E A R G A U F U M M I
O E H R R T F L I Y U G X L O N
K L R I N Q P K Z P N K A L A C
U W E O C K L Q H L V R K A G R
E S R N Z G V E T D D H V O T O
L F B L O O D H R Q E Y U R P T
```

essential
experience
10

Word Search—Circulatory System

After determining the correct word from the clues provided, locate the words in the word search puzzle.

Word	Clue
_____	A clear yellowish fluid that carries waste and impurities away from the cells
_____	The fluid part of the blood in which the red and white blood cells and blood platelets flow
_____	Blood circulation that goes from the heart to the lungs to be purified
_____	Artery that supplies the thumb side of the arm and the back of the hand
_____	Carries oxygen to the cells
_____	Artery that supplies the little finger side of the arm and the palm of the hand
_____	Allows blood to flow in only one direction
_____	The circulatory system
_____	Thin-walled blood vessels that are less elastic than arteries
_____	Lower thick-walled chamber of the heart

```
U  B  E  M  B  C  Q  K  P  X  D  M  A  V  V  N
U  L  S  S  P  A  C  R  C  J  D  L  E  O  A  O
B  S  N  U  W  Y  O  Y  Q  Y  I  I  L  S  S  X
W  S  E  A  I  U  O  E  O  M  N  A  E  C  C  K
Q  O  Y  V  R  G  U  V  F  S  I  L  W  P  U  J
X  N  T  R  L  T  H  Y  Y  D  C  M  K  M  L  H
Z  R  S  G  A  A  N  J  A  S  W  M  I  T  A  E
P  W  J  Y  D  N  V  R  U  P  I  I  F  K  R  E
V  I  S  W  P  J  O  P  L  P  F  B  G  D  U  L
E  C  E  V  G  A  R  M  H  W  O  Q  R  D  J  C
T  R  B  Z  H  O  U  X  L  A  H  K  W  F  E  I
D  W  Y  P  C  I  C  J  S  U  M  E  G  H  X  R
U  S  M  D  O  X  S  S  E  H  P  S  Q  O  A  T
N  Y  E  U  D  L  T  E  V  X  R  H  A  S  X  N
L  R  I  K  A  F  D  C  M  Q  G  U  Y  L  E  E
O  T  M  I  F  S  P  C  U  B  D  D  I  P  P  V
```

essential experience 11

Matching Exercise

Match each of the following essential terms with its definition.

_____ Inhalation	**1.** Primary structural unit of the nervous system
_____ Eleventh	**2.** Sensory nerves
_____ Neuron	**3.** The largest of the cranial nerves
_____ Temporal	**4.** Affects the muscles of the temple
_____ Lungs	**5.** Affects the skin of the lower lip and chin
_____ Endocrine	**6.** Branch of anatomy that deals with the nervous system and its disorders
_____ Afferent	**7.** Affects the side of the neck and the platysma
_____ Glands	**8.** Affects the skin between the eyes and upper side of the nose
_____ Kidneys	**9.** Affects the muscles of the neck and back
_____ Fifth cranial	**10.** Specialized organs that vary in size and function
_____ Diaphragm	**11.** Eliminates decomposed and undigested food
_____ Supratrochlear	**12.** Ductless glands
_____ Large intestine	**13.** Eliminates perspiration
_____ Mental	**14.** A muscular wall that controls breathing
_____ Enzymes	**15.** During this, oxygen is absorbed into the blood
_____ Cervical	**16.** These are responsible for the chemical changes in food
_____ Skin	**17.** Excrete urine
_____ Neurology	**18.** Exhale carbon dioxide

essential review

Complete the following review of Chapter 6, "Anatomy and Physiology," by circling the correct answer to each question.

1. The uppermost and largest bone of the arm is the _____ .

   a) humerus   b) radius

   c) ulna   d) metacarpus

2. The structure found in the cell center that plays an important part in cell reproduction is the _____ .

   a) nucleus   b) centrosome

   c) cell membrane   d) nucleolus

3. The involuntary muscles that function automatically are called _____ .

   a) striated   b) striped

   c) nonstriated   d) cardiac

4. To grow and thrive, the cell must receive an adequate supply of food, oxygen, and _____ .

   a) toxins   b) poisons

   c) pressure   d) water

5. A group of cells of the same kind are _____ .

   a) organs   b) tissues

   c) systems   d) groups

6. The artery that supplies the back of the head up to the crown is the _____ .

   a) supra orbital   b) occipital

   c) infra-orbital   d) posterior auricular

7. The process of building up larger molecules from smaller ones is called _____ .

   a) anabolism   b) homeostasis

   c) catabolism   d) secretion

8. The small bone on the thumb side of the forearm is the _____ .

   a) humerus   b) radius

   c) ulna   d) metacarpus

9. The protoplasm is enclosed in the cell _____ .

   a) membrane   b) nucleolus

   c) centrosome   d) cytoplasm

10. The artery that supplies blood to the side of the nose is the _____ .

   a) anterior auricular artery   b) external carotid artery

   c) facial artery   d) angular artery

essential review *continued*

11. The muscle that produces the contour of the front and inner side of the upper arm is called the _____ .

    a) cardiac   b) tricep

    c) biceps   d) epicranius

12. Motor nerves or _____ nerves carry impulses from the brain to the muscle.

    a) efferent   b) mixed

    c) afferent   d) sensory

13. The epicranius consists of two parts: the frontalis and the _____ .

    a) aponeurosis   b) occipito-frontalis

    c) corrugator   d) occipitalis

14. Structures designed to accomplish a specific function are _____ .

    a) organs   b) tissues

    c) systems   d) groups

15. The muscle located behind the ears is the _____ .

    a) auricularis superior   b) auricularis anterior

    c) auricularis posterior   d) zygomaticus

16. The nerve that affects the skin of the forehead, scalp, eyebrow, and upper eyelid is the _____ .

    a) supra trochlear   b) supra orbital

    c) infra trochlear   d) infra orbital

17. The artery that supplies the chin and lower lip is the _____ .

    a) submental   b) inferior

    c) angular   d) superior labial

18. The artery that supplies the scalp, the area back and above the ear, and the skin behind the ear is the _____ .

    a) supra orbital   b) occipital

    c) parietal   d) posterior auricular

19. Cells are made up of a colorless, jellylike substance called _____ .

    a) nucleolus   b) nucleus

    c) protoplasm   d) centrosome

20. The study of the structure of the body and what is it made of is _____ .

    a) physiology   b) histology

    c) anatomy   d) osteology

essential **review** *continued*

21. The _____ system changes food into soluble form, suitable for use by the cells of the body.

a) endocrine

b) respiratory

c) excretory

d) digestive

22. The wrist, or _____ , is a flexible joint composed of eight small, irregular bones.

a) metacarpus

b) ulna

c) carpus

d) digits

23. The _____ vascular system consists of the heart and blood vessels for the circulation of the blood.

a) lymph

b) circulatory

c) lymphatic

d) blood

24. The process of breaking down larger substances or molecules into smaller ones is _____ .

a) anabolism

b) homeostasis

c) catabolism

d) secretion

25. The study of the minute structural parts of the body, such as tissues, hair, nails, sweat glands, and oil glands, is _____ .

a) physiology

b) histology

c) anatomy

d) osteology

26. The fingers, or _____ , consist of three phalanges in each finger and two in the thumb, totaling fourteen bones.

a) metacarpus

b) ulna

c) carpus

d) digits

27. The scientific study of bones, their structure and their functions is _____ .

a) physiology

b) histology

c) anatomy

d) osteology

28. The bone that forms the prominence of the cheeks is the _____ .

a) nasal

b) zygomatic

c) maxillae

d) lacrimal

29. The small fragile bone located at the front part of the inner wall of the eye socket is the _____ .

a) nasal

b) zygomatic

c) maxillae

d) lacrimal

30. The elastic, bony cage that serves as a protective framework for the heart, lungs, and other internal organs is the _____ .

a) sternum

b) clavicle

c) scapula

d) thorax

31. The part of the cell that contains food materials necessary for growth, reproduction, and self-repair is the _____ .

a) cytoplasm

b) centrosome

c) nucleolus

d) cell membrane

32. The _____ system's function is to produce all movements of the body.

a) circulatory

b) skeletal

c) muscular

d) nervous

33. The physical founction of the body is the _____ system.

a) circulatory

b) skeletal

c) muscular

d) nervous

34. Voluntary muscles that are controlled by will are called _____ .

a) striated

b) smooth

c) nonstriated

d) cardiac

35. What bone forms the lower back part of the cranium?

a) parietal

b) temporal

c) frontal

d) occipital

36. The part of the muscle that moves is the _____ .

a) origin

b) belly

c) insertion

d) middle

37. The _____ system is made up of the skin and its various accessory organs.

a) endocrine

b) excretory

c) integumentary

d) reproductive

38. The muscle that completely surrounds the margin of the eye socket is the _____ .

a) corrugator

b) orbicularis oculi

c) procerus

d) orbicularis oris

39. The _____ vertebrae form the top part of the spinal column located in the neck region.

a) cervical

b) thorax

c) hyoid

d) thoracic

essential review *continued*

40. The _____ muscle covers the bridge of the nose.

a) corrugator

b) orbicularis oculi

c) procerus

d) orbicularis oris

41. What bone forms the forehead?

a) parietal

b) temporal

c) frontal

d) occipital

42. The muscle that compresses the cheeks and expels air between the lips, as in blowing, is the _____ .

a) caninus

b) mentalis

c) orbicularis oris

d) buccinator

43. The muscle that forms a flat band around the upper and lower lips is the _____ .

a) caninus

b) mentalis

c) orbicularis oris

d) buccinator

44. The muscle that extends along the side of the chin and draws down the corner of the mouth is the _____ .

a) triangularis

b) risorius

c) zygomaticus

d) masseter

45. The muscles of the upper part of the cheek are affected by the _____ nerve.

a) mandible

b) zygomatic

c) temporal

d) buccal

46. A broad muscle that extends from the chest and shoulder to the side of the chin is the _____ .

a) pectoralis

b) serratus anterior

c) platysma

d) supinators

47. _____ turn(s) the hand outward and palm upward.

a) pectoralis

b) serratus anterior

c) platysma

d) supinators

48. The muscle that straightens the wrist, hand, and fingers to form a straight line is the _____ .

a) opponent

b) adductor

c) extensors

d) abductor

49. The _____ muscles draw the fingers together.

a) opponent

b) adductor

c) extensors

d) abductor

essential review *continued*

50. The _____ system controls and coordinates the functions of all the other systems and makes them work harmoniously.

a) circulatory　　　　　　b) skeletal

c) muscular　　　　　　　d) nervous

51. The _____ and the temporalis coordinate in opening and closing the mouth and are referred to as chewing muscles

a) triangularis　　　　　　b) risorius

c) zygomaticus　　　　　　d) masseter

52. There are three main divisions of the nervous system: the central, the _____ , and the autonomic nervous systems.

a) peripheral　　　　　　　b) sympathetic

c) parasympathetic　　　　d) brain

53. The point and lower side of the nose are affected by the _____ nerve.

a) supra orbital　　　　　　b) supra trochlear

c) nasal　　　　　　　　　d) infra trochlear

54. The _____ nerve affects the muscles of the chin and lower lip.

a) mandible　　　　　　　b) zygomatic

c) temporal　　　　　　　d) buccal

55. The _____ assists in breathing and in raising the arm.

a) pectoralis　　　　　　　b) serratus anterior

c) platysma　　　　　　　d) supinators

56. The _____ occipital nerve is located at the base of the skull, and affects the scalp and muscles of this region.

a) greater　　　　　　　　b) auricular

c) smaller　　　　　　　　d) cervical

57. The smaller nerve that supplies the arm and the hand is the _____ nerve.

a) ulnar　　　　　　　　　b) radial

c) median　　　　　　　　d) digital

58. Sensory nerves, called _____ nerves, carry impulses or messages from the sense organs to the brain.

a) efferent　　　　　　　　b) motor

c) afferent　　　　　　　　d) mixed

essential review *continued*

59. The _____ nerve affects the membrane and skin of the nose.

a) supra orbital

b) supra trochlear

c) nasal

d) infra trochlear

60. The _____ nerve supplies all the fingers of the hand.

a) ulnar

b) radial

c) median

d) digital

61. The lower thick-walled chambers of the heart are the left and right _____ .

a) atria

b) ventricles

c) auricles

d) valves

62. Minute, thin-walled blood vessels that connect the smaller arteries to the veins are the

_____ .

a) arteries

b) veins

c) capillaries

d) blood

63. The _____ system is situated within the chest cavity, which is protected on both sides by the ribs.

a) endocrine

b) respiratory

c) excretory

d) digestive

64. _____ circulation is the blood circulation from the heart throughout the body and back again to the heart.

a) systemic

b) plasma

c) pulmonary

d) platelet

65. The fluid part of the blood in which the red and white blood cells and blood platelets flow is _____ .

a) lymph

b) corpuscles

c) leucocytes

d) plasma

66. The clear yellowish fluid that carries waste and impurities away from the cells is known as

_____ .

a) lymph

b) corpuscles

c) leucocytes

d) plasma

67. The _____ artery supplies the lower lip.

a) submental

b) inferior labial

c) angular

d) superior labial

essential review *continued*

68. The artery that supplies the crown and side of the head is the _____ .

   a) parietal
   b) transverse
   c) temporal
   d) frontal

69. The system that purifies the body by eliminating waste material is the _____ system.

   a) endocrine
   b) respiratory
   c) excretory
   d) digestive

70. The collarbone that joins the sternum and scapula is also called the _____ .

   a) humerus
   b) ulna
   c) radius
   d) clavicle

essential discoveries and accomplishments

In the space below, jot some notes about what concepts of this chapter were hardest for you to understand or remember. Imagine finding yourself suddenly in the role of "teacher" and consider what you would tell your "students" about these difficult concepts.

Share your *Essential Discoveries* with some of the other students in your class and ask if they are helpful to them. You may want to revise your notes based on good ideas shared by your peers. Under "Accomplishments," list at least three things you have accomplished since your last entry that relate to your career goals.

Discoveries:

_____

_____

_____

_____

_____

Accomplishments:

_____

_____

_____

_____

_____

_____

chapter 7

The Basics of Chemistry and Electricity

essential objectives

After studying this chapter and completing the Essential Companion *components, you should be able to:*

1. Explain the difference between organic and inorganic chemistry.

2. Discuss the different forms of matter: elements, compounds, and mixtures.

3. Explain pH and the pH scale.

4. Describe oxidation and reduction (redox) reactions.

5. Define the nature of electricity and the two types of electric current.

6. Describe the four types of electrotherapy and their uses.

7. Explain the electromagnetic radiation and the visible spectrum of light.

8. Describe the types of light therapy and their benefits.

essential chemistry and electricity

Why is a basic knowledge of chemistry and electricity important to my career as a cosmetologist?

When you think about it, chemistry has an important role in every product you use, from the water you use to shampoo hair, to the cosmetics applied when giving a facial, to the chemicals you apply to hair in styling or in chemical re-formation. Many of the services you will provide actually change the hair, skin, and nails chemically, as well as physically. Therefore, it is essential that you have a good working knowledge of chemistry in order to provide the safest and most effective services to your clients.

Electricity is the primary source of energy needed, literally, to run the world and the salon where you will work. Electricity is essential for controlling and maintaining the professional environment in every professional establishment. It is responsible for such things as lighting, ventilation, temperature, and possibly even the hot water you will use. Electricity must be used intelligently and safely. As a professional, you must know how it works in order to maintain a safe environment for yourself, your coworkers, and your clients.

Electricity is critical in the salon for use with blow-dryers, curling irons, lotion heaters, wax heaters, facial equipment, cash registers, telephones, computers, nail drills, and so much more. While it is not necessary for you to become an electrical engineer, it is important that you have a working knowledge of how electricity is created and how it can be used safely in the salon.

essential
concepts of basic chemistry and electricity

What do I need to know about basic chemistry and electricity in order to be successful and more effective as a professional cosmetologist?

Like anatomy and physiology, chemistry may be a somewhat scary subject to you. Think of it this way: Chemistry is simply the study of matter; its composition, structure, and properties; and the changes matter may undergo. You know that matter is anything that occupies space and has weight. Organic chemistry deals with all substances in which carbon is present. That, of course, includes animals, plants, petroleum, soft coal, natural gas, and many artificially prepared substances. Most will burn, but cannot be liquified, even though they will dissolve inorganic solvents.

Inorganic chemistry, however, is the branch of chemistry that deals with all substances that do not contain carbon, such as water, air, iron, lead, minerals, and iodine. These are substances that will not burn and are usually soluble in water. Now, your goal in your training as a cosmetologist is not to become a scientist, but you will nonetheless need to develop a comfort level with the basics and the ability to discuss chemistry in relation to your profession. This will increase your credibility significantly with your clients, especially during the consultation process.

You need to be aware of the two types of electricity, how they are measured, and safety devices pertaining to electricity. You will need to have a working knowledge of the various types of currents that are used in the equipment found in the salon. It might help you to think of electricity in terms of the flow of an electric current. As a flow, an electric current is similar to a flow of water. It has a direction, requires a pathway, and can be stopped and started. While the flow of water can actually help create energy, the electric current *is* a flow of energy. It is this passage of energy that gives electricity powers that can be therapeutic or, if handled incorrectly, potentially dangerous and destructive.

essential concepts of basic chemistry and electricity *continued*

The pathway for an electric current flowing through an appliance is called a circuit, which means that the current makes a kind of circle from its source through a conductor and back to its source again. If the current flows in a circuit constantly in one direction, it is called a **direct current** (DC). Most battery-operated devices use direct current. However, most appliances linked by a wall plug to a regional power system use **alternating current** (AC). In alternating current, the current changes direction in a circuit back and forth many times a second.

The flow of electricity can be stopped by simply breaking the circuit through flipping a switch. When the switch is "on," the circuit is completed and electricity can flow. When the switch is "off," the circuit is broken and electricity cannot flow.

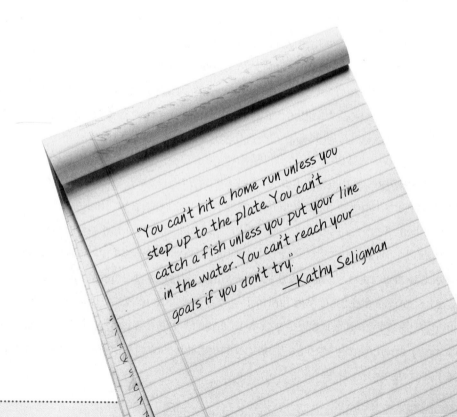

"You can't hit a home run unless you step up to the plate. You can't catch a fish unless you put your line in the water. You can't reach your goals if you don't try."

—Kathy Seligman

essential
1 experience

Organic vs. Inorganic Chemistry

Use your knowledge of the difference between organic and inorganic substances to gather at least ten items in each category. List your items in the space provided and explain what makes them either organic or inorganic.

Organic	Inorganic

essential
experience
2

Product Research

Research a variety of shampoo and conditioning products available in your school, at local supply stores, or at home. Use the chart below to track your findings.

Product Name	Key Ingredients	Purpose of Each Ingredient	Prescribed For Which Hair Type?

essential
3 experience

Matter

In the space below, list examples of how matter can change form. Be specific. For example, when you melt an ice cube (a solid), it becomes water (a liquid), and when you boil it, it becomes steam (a gas). Not all of your examples will include taking on all three forms.

_____

_____

_____

_____

_____

_____

_____

_____

_____

_____

_____

_____

_____

_____

essential
experience
4

Elements

An element is the basic unit of all matter. It is composed of a single part or unit and cannot be reduced to a more simple substance. There are ninety naturally occurring elements. Each element is identified by a letter symbol. The symbols for each element can be obtained by referring to the Periodic Table of Elements found in almost any chemistry textbook. Numbers are used with elements to indicate how many parts are found in a substance made up of those elements. In the chart below, list the symbols for each substance and then explain its composition. (See the example for water.)

Substance	Symbol	Composition
Water	H_2O	Two parts hydrogen and one part oxygen
Ammonia		
Hydrogen Peroxide		
Nitric Acid		
Sodium Hydroxide		
Sodium Chloride		
Hydrogen		
Sulfur		
Nitrogen		
Oxygen		
Carbon		
Iron		
Lead		
Silver		

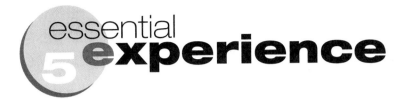

essential experience

Litmus Paper Testing

Obtain a variety of products and test their acidity and alkalinity using litmus paper. List the products you are testing below and state the results. Also, brush one piece of litmus paper with hydrogen peroxide, then brush one half of the litmus paper with a haircolor product. You will actually be able to see the oxidation process take place.

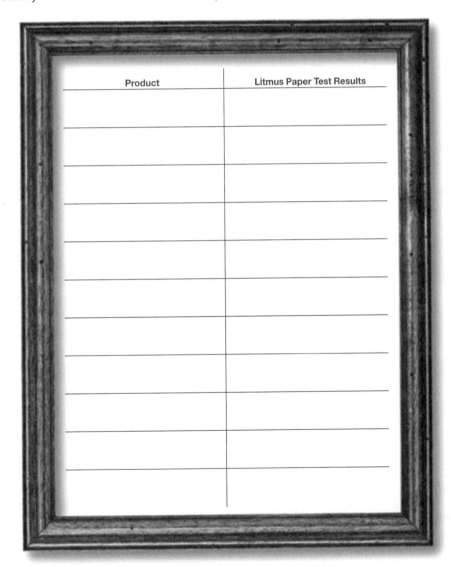

Product	Litmus Paper Test Results

essential
experience
6

Crossword Puzzle

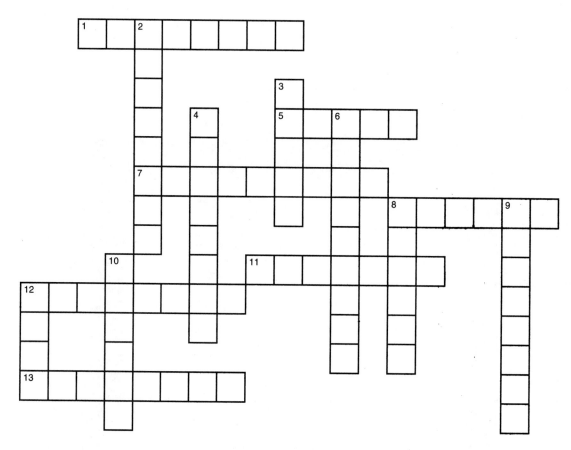

Across

1. Two or more elements chemically joined
5. Compounds of hydrogen, a nonmetal, and some-times oxygen
7. The releasing of oxygen
8. Most abundant element
11. Branch of chemistry that deals with substances in which carbon is present
12. Compounds of hydrogen, a metal, and oxygen
13. Two or more atoms joined together chemically

Down

2. Substances made up of elements combined physically
3. Formed when the hydrogen part of an acid is replaced by a metal
4. Colorless, odorless, and tasteless gas; 1% of the Earth's crust
6. Branch of chemistry that deals with all substances that do not contain carbon
8. Compounds combined with oxygen

9. Basic units of all matter
10. Anything that occupies space
12. Smallest particle of an element

essential experience 7

Word Search

After determining the correct words from the clues provided, locate the words in the word search puzzle.

_____ Solution having a pH below 7.0
_____ Readily evaporating, colorless liquid
_____ Solution having a pH above 7.0
_____ Colorless gas with pungent odor, composed of hydrogen and nitrogen
_____ The smallest particle of an element that still retains the properties of that element
_____ Science that deals with the composition, structures, and properties of matter
_____ Rapid oxidation of any substance
_____ Chemical combination of two or more atoms of different elements
_____ The simplest form of matter
_____ Mixture of two or more immiscible substances united with the aid of a binder or emulsifier
_____ Sweet, colorless, oily substance formed by the decomposition of oils, fats, or fatty acids
_____ Capable of combining with or attracting water
_____ Not capable of being mixed
_____ Capable of combining with or attracting oil
_____ Any substance that occupies space, has physical and chemical properties, and exists in the form of a solid, liquid, or gas
_____ Two or more atoms joined chemically
_____ Chemical reaction that combines an element or compound with oxygen to produce an oxide
_____ Blended mixture of two or more solids, liquids, or gaseous substances
_____ Surface active agent
_____ State in which solid particles are distributed throughout a liquid medium

```
H  C  W  D  G  L  B  W  B  P  I  K  M  A
T  Y  E  I  Y  U  Q  A  L  C  O  H  O  L
C  P  D  L  U  R  E  T  T  A  M  O  L  G
J  Y  S  R  B  L  T  M  P  O  W  M  E  L
N  P  U  N  O  I  T  S  U  B  M  O  C  Y
A  G  S  Q  D  P  C  K  I  L  J  Q  U  C
V  K  P  E  S  O  H  S  Z  M  S  Q  L  E
F  H  E  E  O  P  C  I  I  H  E  I  E  R
A  F  N  K  S  H  C  O  L  M  D  H  O  I
I  O  S  G  U  I  C  T  M  I  M  N  C  N
N  O  I  T  U  L  O  S  C  P  C  I  S  M
O  J  O  O  X  I  D  A  T  I  O  N  R  N
M  T  N  A  T  C  A  F  R  U  S  U  J  E
M  M  K  C  I  R  S  E  L  E  M  E  N  T
A  L  K  A  L  I  B  N  B  A  T  U  B  D
```

essential
experience
8

Word Scramble

Scramble	Correct Word(s)
eotuls	_ _ _ _ _ _ *Clue:* Any substance that dissolves into a liquid and forms a solution
etawr	_ _ _ _ _ *Clue:* A universal solvent
iicilbesmm	_ _ _ _ _ _ _ _ _ _ *Clue:* Not mixable
lelitavo	_ _ _ _ _ _ _ _ *Clue:* Easily evaporated
lnmioseu	_ _ _ _ _ _ _ _ *Clue:* Formed when two or more immiscible substances are united with the aid of a binder
melsbiic	_ _ _ _ _ _ _ _ *Clue:* Mixable
peword	_ _ _ _ _ _ *Clue:* Physical mixture of two solids
setpsa	_ _ _ _ _ _ *Clue:* Semisolid mixture made of petrolatum, oil, and wax
snoituol	_ _ _ _ _ _ _ _ *Clue:* Evenly dispersed mixtures of two or more kinds of molecules
tnevols	_ _ _ _ _ _ _ *Clue:* Any substance that is able to dissolve another substance
iosnnpesus	_ _ _ _ _ _ _ _ _ _ *Clue:* Mixtures of one type of matter in another type of matter
nntsiemto	_ _ _ _ _ _ _ _ _ *Clue:* Semisolid mixtures of organic substances and a medicinal agent

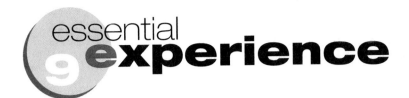

Matching Exercise

Match the following essential terms with their identifying phrases or definition.

_____ Alcohol

_____ Acid

_____ Ammonia water

_____ Disincrustation

_____ Atom

_____ Glycerine

_____ Petrolatum

_____ Lipophilic

_____ Redox

_____ Silicone

1. Special type of oil used in hair conditioners and as a water-resistant lubricant for the skin.

2. A sweet, colorless, odorless, oily substance formed by the decomposition of oils, fats, or fatty acids.

3. Process used to soften and emulsify grease deposits and blackheads in the hair follicles.

4. Chemical reaction in which the oxidizing agent is reduced and the reducing agent is oxidized.

5. Having an affinity or attraction to fat and oils.

6. Another term for petroleum jelly.

7. The smallest particle of an element that still retains the properties of that element.

8. A colorless liquid with a pungent odor, composed of hydrogen and nitrogen in a water solution.

9. A colorless liquid obtained by the fermentation of starch, sugar, and other carbohydrates.

10. Having a pH below 7.0.

essential
10 experience

Conductors and Types of Electricity

A conductor is a substance that permits electric current to pass through it easily. A nonconductor is a substance that resists the passage of an electric current. Identify all the items listed below as either conductors or nonconductors of electricity by writing a C or N in the space provided.

_____ Dry wood   _____ Silk   _____ Asbestos

_____ Wet cotton   _____ Silver   _____ Tar

_____ Copper   _____ Aluminum   _____ Water

_____ Glass   _____ Rubber   _____ Bricks

_____ Human body   _____ Carbon   _____ Linen

_____ Cement   _____ Acid or salt solutions

Describe the construction of an electric wire:

_____

_____

In your own words, explain the difference between a direct current and an alternating current.

Direct current: _____

_____

_____

Alternating current: _____

_____

_____

Can one type of current be changed into another type? _____ Explain: _____

_____

_____

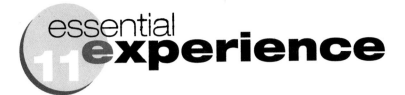

Matching Exercise—Electrical Measurements

Match each of the following essential terms with its definition.

_____ Volt

_____ Amp

_____ Milliampere

_____ Ohm

_____ Watt

_____ Kilowatt

1. Measurement of how much electric energy is being used in one second.

2. 1/1,000 of an ampere. The current for facial and scalp treatments is measured in this manner.

3. The unit of measurement for the strength of an electric current (the number of electrons flowing through a wire).

4. Unit for measuring the pressure that forces the electric current forward.

5. The electricity in your house is measured with this unit.

6. This unit measures the resistance of an electric current. Unless the force is stronger than the resistance, current will not flow through the wire.

essential
12 experience

Safety of Electrical Equipment

Fill in the blanks for the safety precautions that should be followed to avoid accidents and ensure greater client satisfaction.

1. All the electrical appliances you use should be _____ .

2. Read all _____ before using any electrical equipment.

3. _____ all appliances when not in use.

4. _____ all electrical equipment regularly.

5. Keep all wires, plugs, and equipment in good _____.

6. Use only one plug to each _____.

7. You and your client should avoid contact with _____ and metal surfaces when using electricity.

8. Do not leave your client unattended while _____ to an electrical device.

9. Keep electrical cords off the _____ and away from people's feet.

10. Do not attempt to _____ around electric outlets while equipment is plugged in.

11. Do not touch two _____ objects at the same time if either is connected to an electric current.

12. Do not step on or place _____ on electrical cords.

13. Do not allow electrical cord to become _____ as it can cause a short circuit.

14. Disconnect appliances by pulling on the _____, not the cord.

15. Do not attempt to _____ electrical appliances unless you are qualified.

essential experience

13

Crossword Puzzle—Electricity

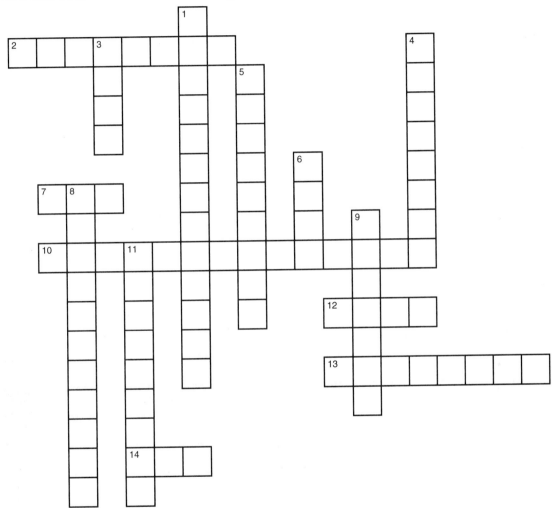

Across

2. Most commonly used modality
7. Unit that measures the strength of an electric current
10. An electronic facial treatment
12. Measurement of how much electric energy is being used in one second
13. Equals 1,000 Watts
14. Unit for measuring resistance of an electric current

Down

1. A constant, even-flowing current, traveling in one direction
3. Unit for measuring the pressure that forces electric current forward
4. Negative or positive state of electric current
5. Nonconductor
6. Safety device that prevents the overheating of electric wires
8. 1/1,000th of an ampere
9. Alternating and interrupted current that produces a mechanical reaction without a chemical effect
11. Substance that permits electric current to pass through it easily

essential
experience
14

The Visible Spectrum

Color in the visible spectrum depicted in the diagram using colored pencils, crayons, or watercolors.

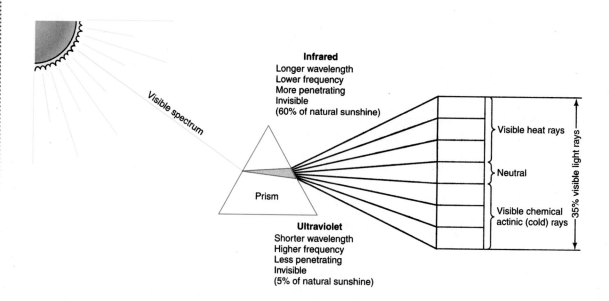

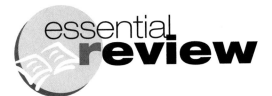

Using the words provided, fill in the blanks below to form a thorough review of Chapter 7, "The Basics of Chemistry and Electricity." Words or terms may be used more than once or not at all.

acid	combustion	hydrophilic	oxidizing
alcohol	compound	infrared	physical
alkaline	conductor	inorganic	polarity
alkanolamines	converter	light rays	radiant energy
alternating	density	lipophilic	rectifier
ampere	direct	liquids	solute
anaphoresis	disincrustation	matter	solvents
anode	electricity	miscible	surfactant
atom	electrode	mixtures	suspension
blue	element	molecule	therapeutic
cathode	emulsions	ointments	vaporizer
chemical	formaldehyde	organic	volatile
chemistry	galvanic	overheating	water
circuit breaker	high-frequency	oxidation	

1. A solution that has a pH less than 7 has an _____ pH, and a solution that has a pH higher than 7 has an _____ pH.

2. A _____ change is a change in the form of a substance, without the formation of a new substance. A _____ change occurs when a new substance is formed.

3. A _____ is a substance that acts as a bridge to allow oil and water to mix, or emulsify.

4. _____ is a readily evaporating, colorless liquid obtained by the fermentation of starch, sugar, and other carbohydrates.

5. An _____ is the smallest particle of an element that is capable of showing the properties of that element.

6. Anything that occupies space is defined as _____.

7. Characteristics of physical properties include _____, specific gravity, hardness, odor, and color.

8. _____ are formed when two or more immiscible substances, such as oil and water, are united with the aid of a binder.

essential review *continued*

9. _____ chemistry is the branch of chemistry that deals with all substances that do not contain carbon.

10. Matter exists in three forms, solids, _____, and gases.

11. _____, pastes, pomades, and styling waxes are semisolid mixtures made with any combination of petrolatum, oil, and wax.

12. _____ chemistry is the branch of chemistry that deals with all substances in which carbon is present.

13. _____ agents are substances that readily release oxygen.

14. Solvents are classified as _____ and immiscible.

15. _____ are any substances that are able to dissolve another substance.

16. Surfactant molecules have two ends: _____ and _____.

17. A _____ is a state in which solid particles are distributed throughout a liquid medium.

18. The universal solvent is _____.

19. The basic unit of all matter is an _____.

20. The science that deals with the composition, structure, and properties of matter is _____.

21. To measure the pH of products, use _____ paper.

22. Two or more atoms that are joined together chemically form a _____.

23. When a substance is made up of two or more different elements, chemically joined, it is a _____.

24. When elements combine physically, they are called _____.

25. When oxygen combines with other substances so rapidly that light energy as well as heat is created, the process is known as _____.

26. _____ is a form of energy that produces magnetic, chemical, and thermal effects.

27. A _____ is a substance that permits electrical current to pass through it easily.

28. A steamer or _____ produces moist, uniform heat that can be applied to the head or face.

29. A _____ is used to change direct current into alternating current, and a _____ is used to change alternating current to direct current.

30. A positive electrode is called a/an _____, and a negative electrode is called a/an _____.

essential review *continued*

31. A fuse is a safety device that prevents the _____ of electric wires.

32. An amp or _____ is the unit that measures the strength of an electric current (the number of electrons flowing through a wire).

33. An _____ is an applicator that directs the electric current from the machine to the client's skin.

34. _____ is the process of forcing liquids into the tissues from the negative toward the positive pole.

35. Artificial light rays are produced by using an electrical apparatus called a _____ lamp.

36. _____ current is a constant, even-flowing current, traveling in one direction, while _____ current is a rapid and interrupted current, flowing first in one direction, then in the opposite.

37. Do not use the negative _____ current on skin with broken capillaries or pustular acne, or on a client with high blood pressure.

38. In modern electric wiring, the fuse has largely been replaced by the _____.

39. _____ rays make up 60 percent of natural sunlight.

40. Therapeutic lamps are used to produce artificial _____ in the salon.

41. The negative or positive state of electric current is _____.

42. The _____ current is characterized by a high rate of oscillation or vibration.

43. The process used to soften and liquify grease deposits in the hair follicles is _____.

44. The _____ light contains few heat rays and has some germicidal and chemical benefits.

45. _____ creates a chemical change in the identity of a substance.

46. The dissolved substance in a solution is known as a _____.

47. _____ alcohols are those that evaporate easily.

48. Substances that are used to neutralize acids or raise the pH of many hair products are known as _____.

49. A preservative used in cosmetics that is toxic to inhale, a strong irritant, and a carcinogenic is _____.

50. Another name for electromagnetic radiation is _____.

essential discoveries and accomplishments

In the space below, jot some notes about what concepts of this chapter were hardest for you to understand or remember. Imagine finding yourself suddenly in the role of "teacher" and consider what you would tell your "students" about these difficult concepts.

Share your *Essential Discoveries* with some of the other students in your class and ask if they are helpful to them. You may want to revise your notes based on good ideas shared by your peers. Under "Accomplishments," list at least three things you have accomplished since your last entry that relate to your career goals.

Discoveries:

_____

_____

_____

_____

_____

Accomplishments:

_____

_____

_____

_____

_____

_____

Properties of the Hair and Scalp

After studying this chapter and completing the Essential Companion *components, you should be able to:*

1. Name and describe the structures of the hair root.

2. List and define the three layers of the hair shaft.

3. List and describe the three types of side bonds in the cortex.

4. List the four factors that should be considered in a hair analysis.

5. Describe the process of growth.

6. Discuss the different types of hair loss and their causes.

7. Describe the various options for hair loss treatment.

8. Recognize hair and scalp disorders commonly seen in the salon and school and know which can be treated there.

essential
properties of the
hair and scalp

How will knowing about the underlying properties of the hair and scalp help me to be a more successful cosmetologist?

Men and women of all ages want healthy, attractive hair. As a licensed cosmetology professional, you will be called upon to advise all your clients on the best care and treatment of their hair both inside and outside the professional establishment. In order to provide the best possible counsel to your clients, you must have a thorough understanding of the hair and how it can be damaged. Hair is composed of different layers which are responsible for specific hair qualities. It is essential for you to be able to analyze a client's hair, determine what type of damage the hair has experienced, and properly prescribe corrective treatments. None of these tasks will be possible without your knowledge of the various properties of the hair and scalp.

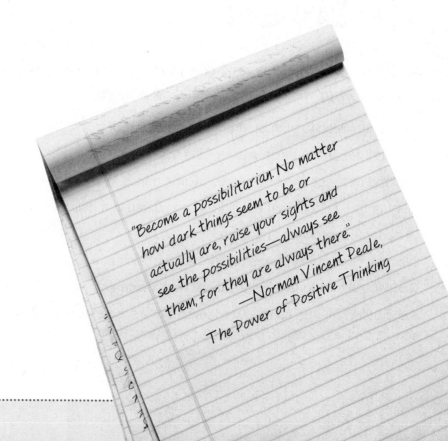

"Become a possibilitarian. No matter how dark things seem to be or actually are, raise your sights and see the possibilities—always see them, for they are always there."
—Norman Vincent Peale,
The Power of Positive Thinking

essential **concepts**

What are the key concepts a professional cosmetologist must understand in order to properly analyze a client's hair and prescribe appropriate corrective treatments?

Trichology is the technical term for the study of hair. As you proceed through your study of trichology, you will gain important insights into how the hair is distributed over the body and the scalp. You will learn that hair is composed chiefly of the protein called keratin and there are two principal parts of hair: the hair root and the hair shaft. As well as understanding the structure of the hair, you will learn how hair grows. Most importantly, however, you will learn to use the senses of sight, touch, hearing, and smell to analyze the condition of a client's hair. Key elements in hair analysis include several hair qualities including texture, porosity, and elasticity. You will also determine that effective scalp manipulation on a regular basis will stimulate the muscles and nerves of the scalp as well as increase the blood circulation in the scalp area.

Another important area of awareness is that of hair loss, which affects over 63 million people in the United States. This particular malady can range from the most common type of hair loss, androgenetic alopecia, which is a result of progressive shrinking or miniaturization of certain scalp follicles, to postpartum alopecia, which is a temporary hair loss after pregnancy. The professional cosmetologist must also be able to identify various diseases and disorders of the hair and scalp. This is important because cosmetologists are not allowed to treat certain conditions which must be referred to a medical professional for treatment.

essential
1 experience

Hair Purpose

In your own words, explain the purpose of the two main types of hair found on the body: vellus and terminal hair.

VELLUS: _____

_____

_____

_____

_____

TERMINAL: _____

_____

_____

_____

essential ✚xperience
2

Hair Follicle Structure

Using the following key, please label the cross-section of the hair.

arrector pili	epidermis	sebaceous or oil glands
bulb	hair follicle	
dermal papilla	hair root	

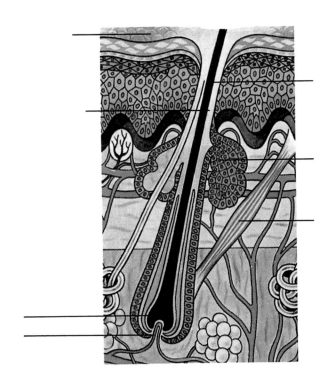

essential
experience
3

Hair Replacement and Growth

Hair growth occurs in cycles. Each complete cycle has three phases that are repeated over and over again throughout life. The three phases are anagen, catagen, and telogen. In your own words, please explain each phase.

ANAGEN: _____

_____

_____

_____

CATAGEN: _____

_____

_____

_____

TELOGEN: _____

_____

_____

_____

essential
4 experience

Directional Hair Growth

Find two individuals with distinct and different hair growth patterns. Diagram the growth patterns using the following head outlines.

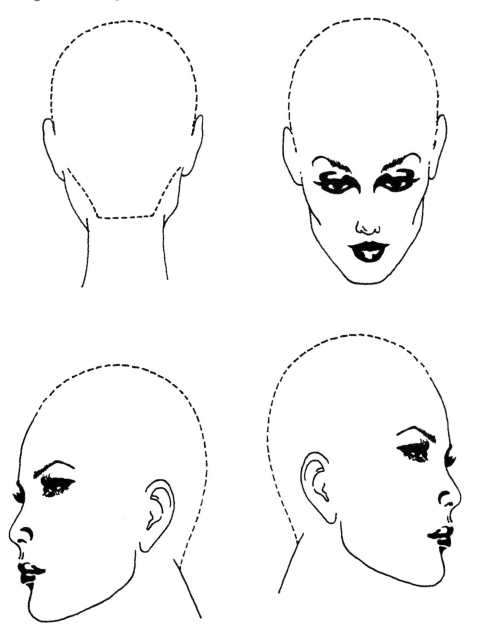

essential experience
5

Word Search—Properties of the Hair and Scalp

After determining the correct words from the clues provided, locate the words in the word search puzzle.

_____	Abnormal hair loss
_____	Growth phase in the hair cycle in which new hair is synthesized
_____	The lowest area or part of a hair strand
_____	The technical term for gray hair
_____	Result of an acute staphylococci infection; larger than a furuncle
_____	Transitional phase of hair growth
_____	Middle layer of the hair
_____	Outermost layer of hair
_____	The number of hairs per square inch on the scalp
_____	Chemical side bond that joins the sulfur atoms of two neighboring cysteine amino acids to create cystine
_____	The ability of the hair to stretch and return to its original length
_____	Tubelike depression, or pocket, in the skin or scalp that contains the hair root
_____	Combined with *crinium,* it's the technical term for brittle hair
_____	Innermost layer of hair
_____	Technical term for beaded hair
_____	Dandruff
_____	The ability of the hair to absorb moisture
_____	The part of the hair structure found below the skin surface
_____	Skin disease caused by the itch mite
_____	Dry, sulfur-yellow, cuplike crusts on the scalp in tinea favosa or favus
_____	The portion of the hair that projects beyond the skin
_____	The thickness or diameter of the individual hair strand
_____	Ringworm
_____	Hair that forms in a circular pattern, as on the crown

```
L A I C E P O L A A N T S O S I
M Y C A R B U N C L E E I A O N
L L T A X E T R O C U F G D U E
B T S I B P N I F R C T I A M A
O G A I C I O G N A O S U Y N E
N H T L A I S R N R U S T C N A
T R I R T A T I O L I I I F S I
E A L O A I T S F S S E C O E B
X E I H G I R I A N I U O L I U
T N G W E T D I E L T T A L B L
U A A S N E R D U I E E Y I A B
R A R L B Y U O C T N B E C C L
E C F O T B L L O I L O S L S E
E P N I C T E E T T I S S E T N
F D P T U M E D U L L A N I S A
S H A F T X I R H T E L I N O M
```

essential
experience
6

Crossword Puzzle—Properties of the Hair and Scalp

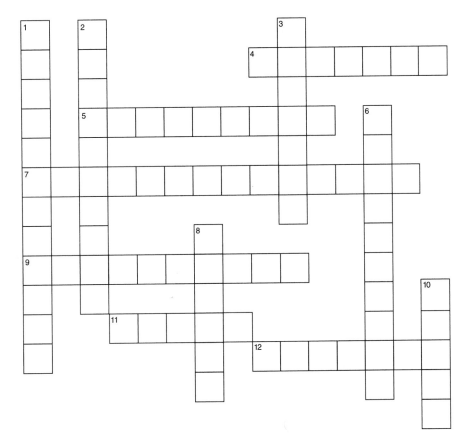

Across

4. Pigment in hair
5. Oil glands
7. Split ends
9. Dandruff
11. Fatty secretion
12. Transitional phase of hair growth

Down

1. Small involuntary muscle
2. Ability of hair to stretch and return to original length
3. Innermost layer of hair
6. Technical term for the study of hair
8. Vellus hair
10. Ringworm

essential 7experience

Grouping Properties of the Hair and Scalp by Category

Place the following terms or procedures into the appropriate category in the chart.

Alopecia areata	Finasteride	Pityriasis steatoides
Anagen	Fine	Porosity
Androgenic alopecia	Follicle	Postpartum alopecia
Arrector Pili	Fragilitas crinium	Scabies
Bulb	Hair root	Telogen
Canities	Hair stream	Texture
Catagen	Hypertrichosis	Tinea
Cortex	Keratin	Tinea capitis
Cowlick	Medulla	Tinea favosa
Cuticle	Minoxidil	Trichoptilosis
Dandruff	Monilethrix	Trichorrhexis nodosa
Density	Pediculosis capitis	Vellus hair
Dermal papilla	Pityriasis	Whorl
Elasticity	Pityriasis capitis simplex	

Hair Distribution, Composition, and Structure:
Hair Growth:
Hair Analysis:
Hair Loss:
Hair Disorders:
Scalp Disorders:

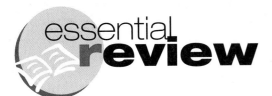

Using the following words, fill in the blanks below to form a thorough review of Chapter 8, "Properties of the Hair and Scalp." Words or terms may be used more than once.

80 percent	cortex	miniaturized	staphylococci
90 percent	cuticle	monilethrix	steatoides
acidic	dandruff	nodular	surface cells
alkaline	disulfide	one-half	swelling
amino acids	elasticity	oval	terminal
androgenic	follicle	pediculosis	three
alopecia	hair bulb	polypeptide	topical
arrector pili	hair root	porosity	trichology
boil	hair shaft	round	trichoptilosis
brittle	hair stream	scabies	unpigmented
canities	healthy diet	scutula	vellus
carbuncle	hydrogen	sebaceous	
cells	hypertrichosis	sebum	
chemicals	lanugo	simplex	

1. The study of the hair is technically called _____.

2. The technical term for the hair found on the face is _____ or lanugo.

3. One basic requisite for healthy hair is a _____.

4. Full-grown human hair is divided into two principal parts, which are known as the hair root and the _____.

5. The two most common types of _____ infections are furuncles and carbuncles.

6. The technical term for hair found on the head is _____ hair.

7. A tube-like depression or pocket in the skin or scalp that encases the hair root is called the _____.

8. The thickened, club-shaped structure that forms the lower part of the hair root is known as the _____.

9. The small involuntary muscle attached to the underside of the hair follicle is called the _____.

essential
review *continued*

10. Fear or the cold causes the _____ to contract, which makes the hair stand up straight, giving the appearance of "goose bumps."

11. Oil glands, which consist of a sac-like structure in the dermis, are also called _____ glands.

12. An oily substance secreted from the sebaceous glands which keeps the skin surface soft and supple is _____ .

13. Hair is composed of cells arranged in _____ layers.

14. The outermost layer of the hair is called the _____ .

15. The cuticle layer of the hair can be raised by _____ .

16. The _____ is the middle layer of the hair which gives it elasticity.

17. The _____ is that portion of the hair that projects beyond the skin.

18. The_____ is that portion of the hair that is located below the surface of the scalp.

19. Another name for vellus hair is _____ .

20. The average growth of healthy hair on the scalp is about _____ inch per month.

21. Hair flowing in the same direction is known as _____ .

22. Cross-sections of straight hair tend to be _____ .

23. Cross-sections of wavy hair are usually _____ .

24. Cross-sections of extremely curly hair tend to be highly_____ .

25. Qualities by which human hair is analyzed are texture, density,_____ , and _____ .

26. The ability of the hair to stretch and return to its original form is _____ .

27. The ability of the hair to absorb moisture is known as_____ .

28. Hair is composed of protein that grows from_____ originating within the hair follicle.

29. Hair is approximately _____ protein.

30. The technical term for the most common type of hair loss is _____ .

31. Hair protein is made up of long chains of _____ which are made up of elements.

essential review *continued*

32. A long chain of amino acids linked by peptide bonds is called a _____ chain.

33. A _____ bond is a physical side bond that is easily broken by water or heat.

34. Minoxidil is a _____ medication applied to the scalp twice daily to stimulate hair growth.

35. The technical term for gray (unpigmented) hair is _____.

36. Salt bonds are easily broken by strong _____ or _____ solutions.

37. An abnormal development of hair on areas of the body that normally bear only downy hair is known as _____ or hirsuties.

38. The technical term for split hair ends is _____.

39. Trichorrhexis nodosa, or knotted hair, is the dry, brittle condition including formation of _____ swellings along the hair shaft.

40. The technical term for beaded hair is _____, which may be improved with scalp and hair treatments.

41. Fragilitas crinium is the technical term for _____ hair that may split at any part of its length.

42. A _____ bond joins the sulfur atoms of two neighboring amino acids.

43. Pityriasis is the medical term for _____.

44. A direct cause of dandruff is the excessive shedding of the scalp's _____.

45. The two principal types of dandruff are pityriasis capitis _____ (the dry type) and pityriasis _____ (the greasy or waxy type).

46. Honeycomb ringworm is characterized by dry, sulfur-yellow, cup-like crusts on the scalp called _____.

47. _____ is a highly contagious, animal parasitic skin disease caused by the itch mite.

48. A contagious condition caused by the head louse is _____ capitis.

49. A furuncle, or _____, is an acute staphylococci infection of a hair follicle.

50. A _____ is the result of an acute staphylococci infection and is larger than a furuncle.

essential discoveries and accomplishments

In the space below, jot some notes about what concepts of this chapter were hardest for you to understand or remember. Imagine finding yourself suddenly in the role of "teacher" and consider what you would tell your "students" about these difficult concepts.

Share your *Essential Discoveries* with some of the other students in your class and ask if they are helpful to them. You may want to revise your notes based on good ideas shared by your peers. Under "Accomplishments," list at least three things you have accomplished since your last entry that relate to your career goals.

Discoveries:

_____

_____

_____

_____

_____

Accomplishments:

_____

_____

_____

_____

_____

_____

Principles of Hair Design

essential **objectives**

After studying this chapter and completing the Essential Companion *components, you should be able to:*

1. List the five elements of hair design.

2. List the five principles of hair design.

3. Identify different facial shapes.

4. Demonstrate how to design hairstyles to enhance or camouflage facial features.

5. Explain design considerations for men.

essential artistry in hairstyling

Why is understanding the basic elements of design so important to my success as a cosmetologist?

The answer is as simple as cooking! If you've ever created a masterpiece in the kitchen or even observed a great cook like your mother or grandmother in action, you know that it takes a great deal more than just knowing what the ingredients are. You must know exactly what quantity of each ingredient is needed. You must know at exactly what point each ingredient is added. You need to know things like cooking temperatures and how to use special kitchen tools such as knives or wire whisks. The exact same principles apply in hairstyling. You must attain a thorough knowledge of all the tools and implements required in creating a great design. In addition, you must know the principles of design and also understand how the client's face shape and features impact the chosen design. Once you have gained a solid working knowledge of all these parts, pieces, and principles, you will be able to provide quality services to each and every client.

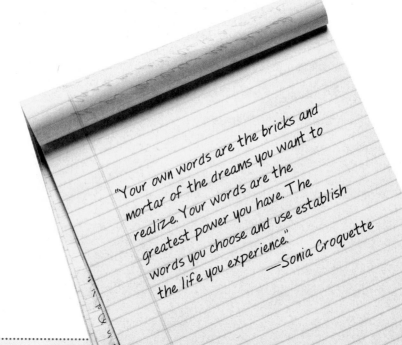

"Your own words are the bricks and mortar of the dreams you want to realize. Your words are the greatest power you have. The words you choose and use establish the life you experience."

—Sonia Croquette

essential design concepts

If there are so many key "ingredients" to hair design, where do I begin?

You must first gain an understanding of the five elements of design: form, space, line, color, and wave pattern. Then you must experiment with those five elements to create a variety of designs. You must also gain knowledge of the principles of hair design, which include proportion, balance, rhythm, emphasis, and harmony, and how each affects the end result. Finally, you must learn about all the client's personal circumstances that will impact the overall design. These include the client's face shape, facial features, head shape, profile, and whether or not the client wears eyeglasses. All of these concepts will be contributing factors as to whether you provide the client with a flattering and satisfactory hair design.

essential
experience
1

The Elements of Design

Form

Take pictures of the same hairstyle on a client or another student from three different angles. Cut around the perimeter of the hairstyle for each angle and, in the area provided below, outline the style in the *Essential Companion*. Discuss with fellow students how different the silhouette is from different angles. (If a camera is not available for your use, be creative. Create a silhouette on a chalkboard in the classroom by adjusting the overhead lighting and using a flashlight or spotlight. Once you've traced three different silhouettes on the chalkboard, copy a smaller version below).

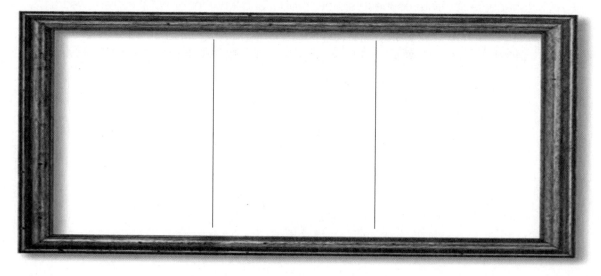

Space

In order to get a better grasp of what is meant by volume and how the same amount of volume can take on a variety of three-dimensional shapes and styles, try this project. At home in your kitchen, measure out exactly eight ounces of water and pour it into a round plastic cup. Measure another eight ounces of water and pour it into a square plastic container. Measure another eight ounces of water and pour it into a rectangular-shaped plastic container. Place all three containers in the freezer. After they are frozen, remove the frozen masses from their respective containers and compare their shapes. Remember, each ice mold represents the exact same volume of water. *Note:* You can use any size or shape of container for this experiment as long as it is freezer safe.

essential experience *continued*

1

Line

Curly, straight, or curved lines create the form, design, and movement of a hairstyle. Depict the following different lines by cutting pictures out of magazines and pasting them in the space provided below. Using a colored pen, emphasize the type of line the style depicts.

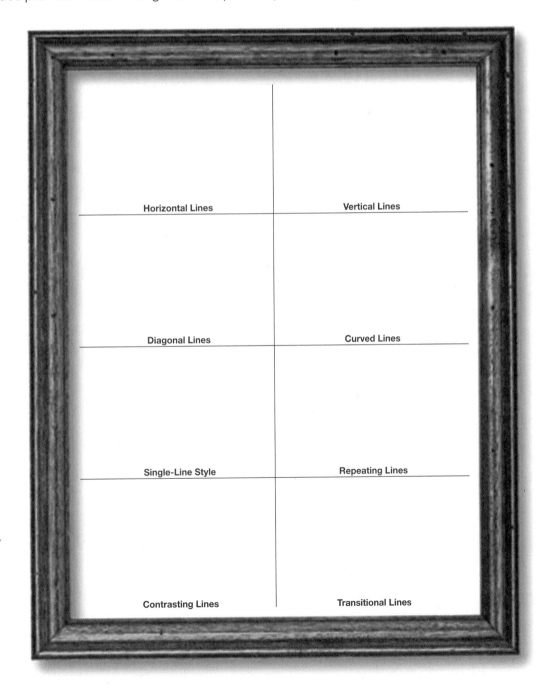

Horizontal Lines	**Vertical Lines**
Diagonal Lines	**Curved Lines**
Single-Line Style	**Repeating Lines**
Contrasting Lines	**Transitional Lines**

essential
experience *continued*

1

Color

You will learn to use color to bring dimension and finish to a style. Think about a living room that is painted a dull beige with a beige carpet and a light brown sofa. It likely appears rather dull. Imagine what a difference you could make if you painted one wall a brighter contrasting color, placed several throw pillows in a variety of textures and colors on the sofa, or added a brightly colored throw rug over the carpet. Imagine the difference any one of those changes would make to the room's overall appearance. The same principle applies to haircolor. Again, using your favorite magazines, select several pictures of different hairstyles and paste them below. Indicate which styles are improved because of color and which ones are just colored for the sake of color or to be different.

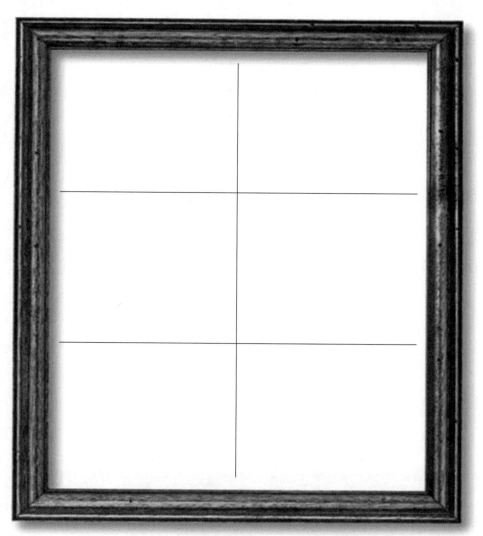

essential experience *continued*

Wave Pattern

All of us have a natural wave pattern. It may be straight, wavy, curly, or extremely curly. When aiding our clients in selecting a hairstyle that will be flattering and easy to maintain, we must take their wave pattern into consideration. In this activity, search magazines for pictures that depict various types of wave patterns. Paste them in the spaces provided below and write a brief explanation about the look created by each wave pattern.

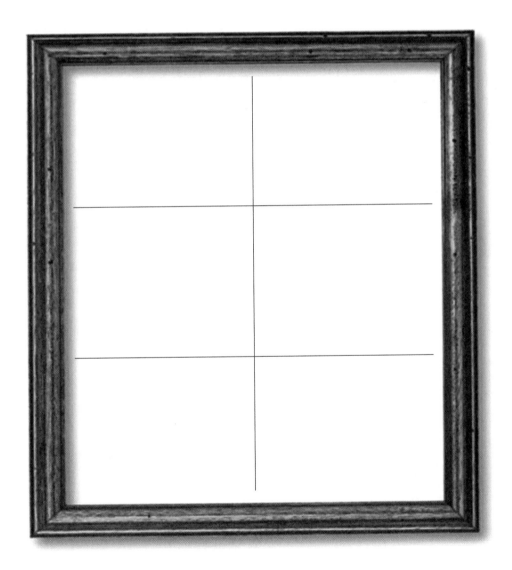

essential
2 experience

The Principles of Design

Proportion

Proportion deals with the harmonious relationship of the parts of something to each other or to the whole. Have you ever seen something that's clearly out of proportion with its surroundings? Perhaps you've observed a cute but extremely tiny foreign car pull into the parking lot at the mall and then watched as a very large man, about six feet six inches tall and 230 pounds, hoisted himself out of the vehicle. He and the car aren't really in harmony with each other. The same principle applies in hair design. This exercise will help you understand the importance of proportion with the face, features, head shape, and body size and shape. Remember, proper proportions are three parts hair to two parts face.

Using poster board or construction paper, paste pictures from magazines which depict the following:

1. Someone whose hairstyle is much too large for a petite body.

2. Someone whose hairstyle is much too small for a larger body frame.

3. Someone whose hairstyle reflects pleasing proportions to the face.

4. Someone whose hairstyle reflects hair out of proportion to the face.

essential
2 experience *continued*

Balance

By balance we mean that the hairstyle is equal in size or volume around the head. It can be either symmetrical or asymmetrical. Sketch the essential concepts of balance in the windowpane spaces below.

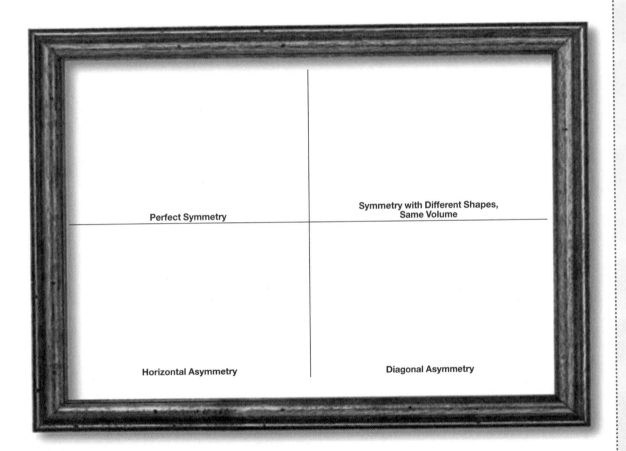

Perfect Symmetry

Symmetry with Different Shapes, Same Volume

Horizontal Asymmetry

Diagonal Asymmetry

Rhythm

When you think of someone having great rhythm, you are likely visualizing how that person moves on a dance floor. Rhythm means the same thing in a hairstyle: movement. Cut six different pictures out of magazines and paste them below. Indicate whether the style has fast or slow rhythm.

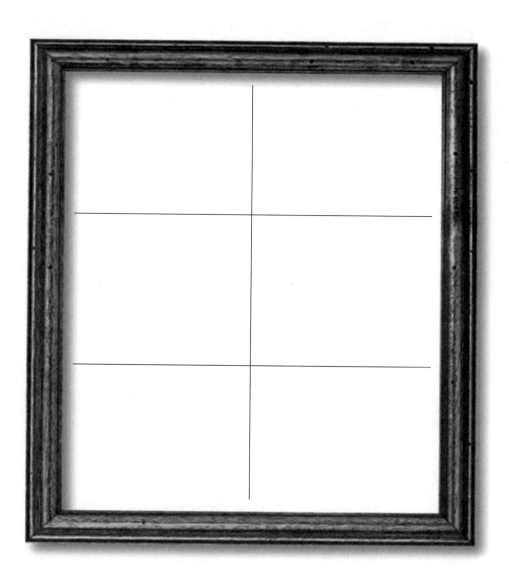

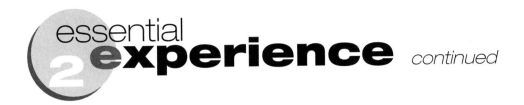

Emphasis

Emphasis is the focal point or the point of prominence in a hairstyle. Our eyes tend to see this part of the style first. List a few ideas about how you can add emphasis to a hairstyle.

_____

_____

_____

_____

_____

Harmony

Without harmony, none of the other principles of design will work. Harmony is what brings a systematic arrangement of all the parts and other principles. Think about anyone you've known, a celebrity perhaps, who may have had great color or balance but the harmony just did not happen. List their names here and explain why there was no harmony.

_____

_____

_____

_____

essential
3 experience

Windowpaning—Facial Types

Windowpaning is the process of transferring key elements, points, or steps in a lesson into visual images that are hand sketched into the squares of "panes" of a matrix. Look through magazines and find pictures that depict the face shapes indicated below. Let your mind think in pictures and sketch the essential concepts printed in each of the following windowpanes.

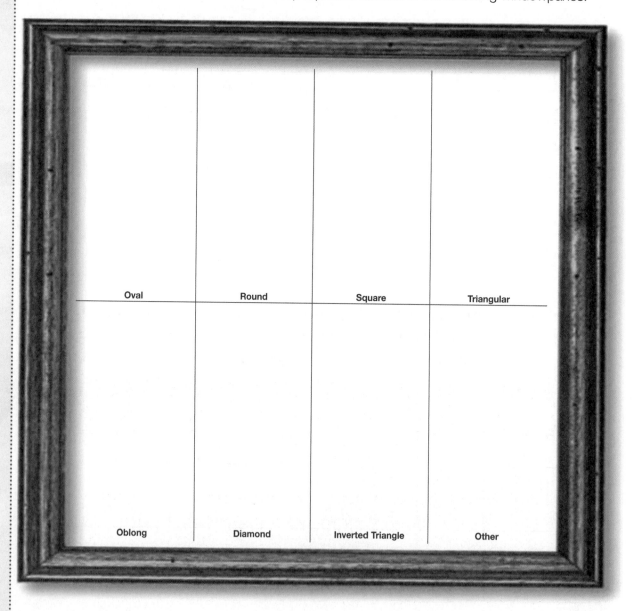

Oval	Round	Square	Triangular
Oblong	Diamond	Inverted Triangle	Other

On a separate sheet of paper, describe the appropriate hairstyle for each face shape in the matrix. In the case of magazine pictures, explain why the hairstyle works or doesn't work.

essential
4 experience

Special Considerations

Match the following essential terms with their identifying terms or phrases by placing the identifying number next to the appropriate term.

_____ Wide forehead

_____ Narrow forehead

_____ Close-set eyes

_____ Wide-set eyes

_____ Crooked nose

_____ Wide, flat nose

_____ Round jaw

_____ Square jaw

_____ Long jaw

_____ Straight profile

_____ Convex profile

_____ Concave profile

_____ Receding forehead

_____ Large forehead

_____ Small nose

_____ Prominent nose

_____ Receding chin

_____ Small chin

_____ Large chin

_____ Triangular part

_____ Diagonal part

_____ Curved part

_____ Side parts

_____ Center parts

_____ Diagonal back parts

_____ Zigzag parts

1. Usually used for an oval face, or to give an oval illusion to wide and round faces

2. Create a dramatic effect

3. Direct hair forward over the sides of the forehead

4. Asymmetrical, off-center styles are best

5. Direct hair back and away from the face at temples; some height is advisable

6. Draw hair away from the face; use center part to elongate

7. Direct fringe over forehead with an outwardly directed volume

8. Sweep hair off face, creating a line from the nose to ear

9. Hair should be shorter or longer than the chin

10. Bring hair forward at the forehead with softness around the face

11. All hairstyles are flattering to this profile

12. Use fringe with little or no volume

13. Arrange curls or bangs over forehead; keep style close to head at nape and move forward toward chin

14. Use straight lines at the jawline

15. Direct hair away from the face at forehead; use light highlights at temples

16. Use half-fringe to create length; darken hair at sides

17. Use curved lines at jawline

essential
4 **experience** *continued*

18. Hair should be full and fall below jawline

19. Hair at nape should be styled softly, with upward movement; don't build hair onto forehead

20. Gives height and width to a round or square face

21. Used for a receding hairline or high forehead

22. Used to direct hair across the top of the head and help develop height

23. Used to create the illusion of width or height

24. The basic parting for fringe sections

essential experience

5

Crossword Puzzle—Artistry in Hairstyling

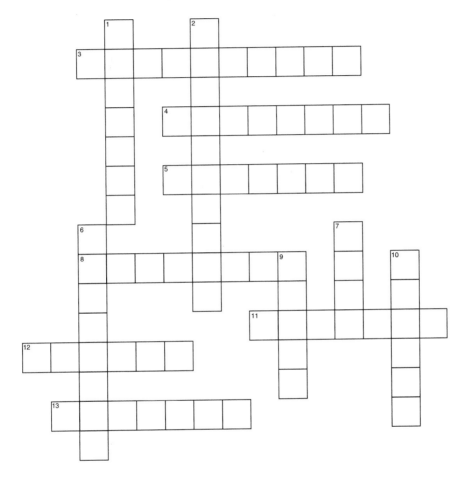

Across

3. Harmonious relationship between parts of things
4. Positioned between horizontal and vertical
5. Curving inward
8. The place the eye turns first in a hairstyle
11. Orderly and pleasing arrangement of shapes and lines
12. Triangular section that begins at apex and ends at front corners
13. Proper degree of height and width

Down

1. Outline of a figure from a side view
2. Parallel to the floor or horizon
6. Lines that are straight up and down
7. The outline of the overall hairstyle
9. The area that the hairstyle occupies
10. Curving outward

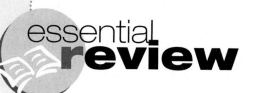
essential
review

Complete the following review of Chapter 9, "Principles of Hair Design," by circling the correct answer to each question.

1. The outline or silhouette of a hairstyle is known as the _____.

    a) space   b) line

    c) form   d) design

2. The form, design, and movement of a hairstyle is created by the _____.

    a) space   b) lines

    c) form   d) design

3. The area that hairstyle occupies is called its volume or _____.

    a) space   b) lines

    c) form   d) design

4. Lines that are parallel to the floor are known as _____.

    a) vertical   b) diagonal

    c) horizontal   d) curved

5. Lines used to soften a design are _____.

    a) vertical   b) diagonal

    c) horizontal   d) curved

6. Lines used to make a hairstyle appear longer and narrower are _____.

    a) vertical   b) diagonal

    c) horizontal   d) curved

7. Lines positioned between horizontal and vertical which are used to create interest are _____.

    a) vertical   b) diagonal

    c) horizontal   d) curved

8. An example of a line that is found in the blunt or one-length hairstyle cut is the _____ line.

    a) single   b) contrasting

    c) transitional   d) repeating

9. Lines that meet at a 90-degree angle and create a hard edge are called _____ lines.

    a) single   b) contrasting

    c) transitional   d) repeating

essential review *continued*

10. Curved lines used to soften and blend horizontal or vertical lines are known as
_____ lines.

a) vertical   b) contrasting

c) transitional   d) repeating

11. Lighter and warmer colors are used to create the illusion of _____.

a) subtlety   b) repetition

c) volume   d) closeness

12. Dark and cool colors move forward or toward the head and create the illusion of less
_____.

a) volume   b) height

c) width   d) strength

13. When choosing haircolor, it should be compatible with the client's _____.

a) eye color   b) skin tone

c) family's choice   d) childhood dreams

14. Wave patterns can be natural or created with styling techniques, chemical changes,
curling irons or _____.

a) client's desire   b) stylist's desire

c) hair brushing   d) hot rollers

15. Curly hair can be permanently straightened with _____.

a) curling irons   b) hair relaxers

c) pressing irons   d) crimping irons

16. Curly and extremely curly hair do not reflect much light and could be _____
to the touch.

a) soft   b) smooth

c) limp   d) coarse

17. The five principles of hair design are proportion, balance, rhythm, emphasis, and
_____.

a) symmetry   b) asymmetry

c) harmony   d) diagonal

18. _____ wave patterns accent the face and are particularly useful when you
wish to narrow a round head shape.

a) rough   b) busy

c) smooth   d) numerous

essential review *continued*

19. The harmonious arrangement of the hair is known as _____.

   a) balance   b) harmony

   c) rhythm   d) emphasis

20. The pattern that creates movement in a hairstyle is known as _____.

   a) balance   b) harmony

   c) rhythm   d) emphasis

21. _____ is considered the most important of the principles of hair design.

   a) balance   b) harmony

   c) rhythm   d) emphasis

22. The _____ in a hairstyle is the place the eyes see first.

   a) balance   b) harmony

   c) rhythm   d) emphasis

23. Generally, the ideal face shape is said to be the _____ shape.

   a) square   b) round

   c) oval   d) pear

24. The face is divided into _____ zones.

   a) one   b) two

   c) three   d) four

25. Creating the illusion of width in the forehead would be best for the _____ face shape.

   a) round   b) triangular

   c) oblong   d) diamond

26. The aim of reducing the width across the cheekbone line is best for the _____ face shape.

   a) round   b) triangular

   c) oblong   d) diamond

27. The aim of making the face appear shorter and wider is best for the _____ face shape.

   a) round   b) triangular

   c) oblong   d) diamond

28. Directing the hair away from the face at the forehead would be best for _____.

   a) a wide forehead   b) close-set eyes

   c) a narrow forehead   d) wide-set eyes

29. Directing the hair forward over the sides of the forehead is best for _____.

    a) a wide forehead

    b) close-set eyes

    c) a narrow forehead

    d) wide-set eyes

30. Asymmetrical, off-center styles are best for _____.

    a) narrow forehead

    b) close eyes

    c) long jawline

    d) crooked nose

31. The profile which has an exaggerated outward curvature is called the _____ profile.

    a) convex

    b) concave

    c) straight

    d) curved

32. The profile which has an inward curvature is called the _____ profile.

    a) convex

    b) concave

    c) straight

    d) curved

33. Bangs with little or no volume should be used for a _____.

    a) receding forehead

    b) large forehead

    c) low forehead

    d) small forehead

34. A part that helps develop height on top and make thin hair appear fuller is the _____ part.

    a) center

    b) side

    c) diagonal

    d) zigzag

35. The _____ part should be used to give height to a round or square face and width to a long thin face.

    a) triangular

    b) diagonal

    c) side

    d) zigzag

36. The _____ part creates what is considered to be a dramatic styling effect.

    a) triangular

    b) diagonal

    c) side

    d) zigzag

37. The _____ part is considered to be the basic parting for the bang section.

    a) triangular

    b) diagonal

    c) side

    d) zigzag

38. The _____ part is used to direct hair across the top of the head.

    a) triangular

    b) diagonal

    c) side

    d) center

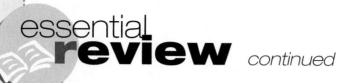

39. The _____ part is considered the classic part and is usually used for an oval face, but can be used to create the illusion of oval for a round or wide face.

a) curved   b) side

c) center   d) diagonal

40. The _____ part is used for a receding hairline or high forehead.

a) curved   b) side

c) center   d) diagonal

essential discoveries and accomplishments

In the space below, jot some notes about what concepts of this chapter were hardest for you to understand or remember. Imagine finding yourself suddenly in the role of "teacher" and consider what you would tell your "students" about these difficult concepts.

Share your *Essential Discoveries* with some of the other students in your class and ask if they are helpful to them. You may want to revise your notes based on good ideas shared by your peers. Under "Accomplishments," list at least three things you have accomplished since your last entry that relate to your career goals.

Discoveries:

_____

_____

_____

_____

_____

Accomplishments:

_____

_____

_____

_____

_____

Shampooing, Rinsing, and Conditioning

essential objectives

After studying this chapter and completing the Essential Companion *components, you should be able to:*

1. Explain pH and its importance in shampoo selection.

2. Explain the role of surfactants in shampoo.

3. Discuss the uses and benefits of various types of shampoos and conditioners.

4. Perform proper scalp manipulations as part of a shampoo service.

5. Demonstrate proper shampoo procedure.

6. Demonstrate proper conditioning procedures.

7. Describe general hair and scalp treatments.

essential shampooing and conditioning

Why are shampooing and conditioning so important to my training when they seem to be such insignificant services?

Just because you have been shampooing and conditioning your own hair for a number of years does not mean that you have appropriate knowledge to deliver a professional shampoo and conditioning service to your clients. It is necessary to understand that the procedure and various products that you have used at home are likely not professional products and may not be client-oriented. In fact, it is not uncommon for people to choose their shampoo or conditioning treatment based on its fragrance or because talented marketing managers suggest it is beneficial for their hair.

Your ability to provide a thorough and pleasing shampoo is essential. It is generally the first service you provide to a client, and it allows you to begin building a positive client relationship. More importantly, the shampoo service is the most repeated service you can provide to your clients. In most cases, a thorough shampoo will precede a haircut, a style, a color treatment, and any chemical reformation. You can be sure that how well you perform the shampoo service will greatly affect the client's perception of how well you will perform other services they desire. And remember, when you give a good shampoo with a relaxing scalp massage, you lay the groundwork for selling the client many more services both today and in the future.

essential concepts

What do I need to know about shampooing, rinsing, and conditioning in order to provide a quality service?

It may help you to understand some history about cleansing the hair. The word *shampoo* is derived from the Hindu word *champna,* which means to press, knead, or shampoo. History tells us that humans have found many ways to cleanse the body in order to prevent disease. Traditionally, people used natural ingredients to accomplish this, including soapwort which is a plant that produces a lather in water. Near the middle of the twentieth century, however, scientists created chemical ingredients to replace the natural ones. Chemists became aware of the pH (potential hydrogen) level of hair and recognized that products should be created that would maintain the natural pH of the hair.

You will also need to know how important proper brushing is before the shampoo service. You will then need to practice and master the shampoo procedure. Once you have accomplished that, you will want to achieve a keen understanding of the chemistry of shampoos, rinses, and conditioning treatments and the effects that those chemicals have on the hair. As a professional cosmetologist, you actually become your client's hair "physician." Therefore, your knowledge of the effects of various products on the hair is critical in your role as a professional consultant who prescribes treatments for the hair.

"Don't let the fear of the time it will take to accomplish something stand in your way of doing it. The time will pass anyway; we might just as well put that passing time to the best possible use."
—Earl Nightingale

essential
experience
1

Find a partner and do a joint research project on the various shampoo products used in your school. You may want to expand the project by researching the shampoo products you both use at home. Use the following chart to list the types of shampoo, the type of hair they are created for, and the ingredients found in each. After you have collected the data, determine any common ingredients in the products. Finally, obtain some litmus paper and test each product to determine the pH level (level of acidity and alkalinity) of each.

Product Name	Recommended for Which Hair Type	Ingredients	pH Level

After identifying the common ingredients, write a brief explanation of why you believe these ingredients are used in so many shampoo products.

_____

_____

_____

_____

essential
2 experience

Using the pH scale provided below, label the pH levels of the shampoos you researched in Essential Experience #1.

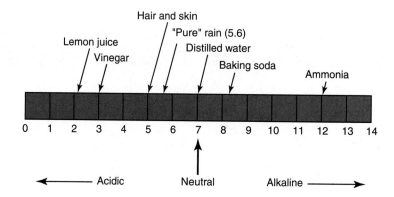

essential
3 experience

Interview senior students or salon professionals and ask them to describe any instances in which they did not properly drape or secure the cape on a client. What were the results of their errors? Record your findings in the space below.

_____

_____

_____

_____

_____

_____

_____

_____

_____

_____

_____

_____

_____

_____

_____

_____

essential
4 experience

Collect hair swatches for various types of hair including normal, color-treated, relaxed, and permed. Shampoo the swatches at least five times with one available shampoo product, using a different shampoo for each swatch. Report the effects of the shampoo on each swatch. Then divide each swatch in half and condition one half. Report on the effects of each shampoo on each swatch. Report on the results after half the swatch has been re-conditioned. Tape the swatches into the box provided.

Swatch Type	Shampoo Used	Results	Conditioned Swatch	Results
Normal				
Color Treated				
Relaxed				
Permed				

Make recommendations for the ideal shampoo for each hair type and explain why others are not appropriate.

_____

_____

_____

essential
experience
5

Arrange to have both soft and hard water available for use for this experiment. Using the different water types and a professional shampoo product, compare the product's lathering ability, cleansing ability, and the appearance of the hair after shampooing. Record your results below.

_____

_____

_____

_____

_____

_____

_____

_____

_____

_____

_____

_____

_____

_____

essential
6 experience

Number the following shampoo scalp manipulations in the order they should occur.

_____ Allow the client's head to relax and work around the hairline with your thumbs in a rotating movement.

_____ Continue in this manner to the back of the head, shifting your fingers back one inch.

_____ Drop your fingers down one inch and repeat the process until the right side of the head is covered.

_____ Begin at the front hairline and work in a back-and-forth movement until the top of the head is reached.

_____ Repeat these movements until the scalp has been thoroughly massaged.

_____ Lift the client's head, with your left hand controlling the movement of the head. With your right hand, start at the top of the right ear and, using the same movement, work to the back of the head.

_____ Remove excess shampoo and lather by squeezing the hair.

_____ Beginning at the left ear, repeat steps 3 and 4.

essential 7 experience

Crossword Puzzle—Shampooing, Rinsing, and Conditioning

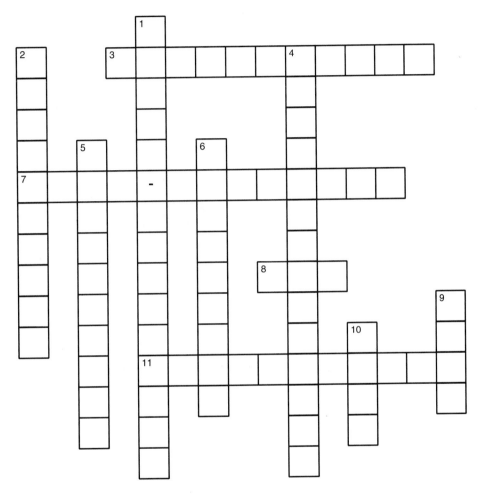

Across

3. Adds moisture to hair
7. Having a balanced pH
8. Shampoo that cleanses without soap and water
11. Moisturizes, restores, and protects hair

Down

1. Shampoo created by combining the surfactant base with basic dyes
2. Detergent
4. Another name for conditioners
5. Attract oil
6. Shampoo that washes away excess oiliness
9. Water containing minerals that lessen the ability to lather
10. Rain water or chemically softened water

essential review

Using the following words, fill in the blanks to form a thorough review of Chapter 10, "Shampooing, Rinsing, and Conditioning." Words or terms may be used more than once or not at all.

0 to 6.9	condition	medicated	shampoos
4.5 to 6.6	dry	natural	skin
7.1 to 14	H_2O	oily	soft
acid	H_2O_2	polymers	stimulating
blood	hard	powder	tangles
brittle	humectants	protein	temperature
chemical service	hydrogen	scales	volume
citric acid	ingredients	shampooing	

1. An important preliminary first step for a variety of hair services is _____.

2. To be effective, a shampoo must remove all dirt, oils, cosmetics, and _____ debris without adversely affecting either the scalp or hair.

3. _____ hair should be shampooed more often than other types.

4. Hair can usually be characterized as oily, _____, normal, or chemically treated.

5. Rain water or water that has been chemically treated is known as _____ water.

6. _____ water contains certain minerals that lessen the ability of the shampoo to lather readily.

7. _____ bristles are recommended for hair brushing.

8. Select the shampoo according to the _____ of the client's hair.

9. A high-pH shampoo can leave the hair dry and _____.

10. You should not brush the hair prior to giving a _____.

11. Brushing stimulates the _____ circulation to the scalp and helps remove dust, dirt, and hair spray buildup from the hair.

12. You should never use the comb to loosen _____ from the scalp.

13. The inner side of your wrist is used to test the water _____.

essential review *continued*

14. Biotin and protein are conditioning agents that restore moisture and elasticity, strengthen the hair shaft, and add _____ .

15. _____ account for the highest dollar expenditure in hair care products.

16. The key to determining which shampoo will leave the hair lustrous and manageable is the _____ list.

17. The amount of _____ in a solution determines whether it is more alkaline or more acid.

18. Shampoos that are more acid fall in the range of _____ on the pH scale.

19. Shampoos that are more alkaline fall in the range of _____ on the pH scale.

20. An acid-balanced shampoo falls in the range of _____ on the pH scale.

21. _____ shampoos contain special chemicals that are effective in reducing excessive dandruff.

22. A dry or _____ shampoo is usually given when the client's health does not permit a regular shampoo.

23. Most conditioners contain silicone along with moisture-binding _____ that absorb moisture or promote the retention of moisture.

24. Penetrating conditioners that are left on the hair for ten to twenty minutes restore _____ and moisture.

25. Emollients reduce frizz and synthetic _____ bulk up the hair.

essential discoveries and accomplishments

In the space below, jot some notes about what concepts of this chapter were hardest for you to understand or remember. Imagine finding yourself suddenly in the role of "teacher" and consider what you would tell your "students" about these difficult concepts.

Share your *Essential Discoveries* with some of the other students in your class and ask if they are helpful to them. You may want to revise your notes based on good ideas shared by your peers. Under "Accomplishments," list at least three things you have accomplished since your last entry that relate to your career goals.

Discoveries:

_____

_____

_____

_____

_____

Accomplishments:

_____

_____

_____

_____

_____

chapter 11

Haircutting

essential **objectives**

After studying this chapter and completing the Essential Companion *components, you should be able to:*

1. Identify reference points on the head form and understand their role in haircutting.

2. Define angles, elevations, and guidelines.

3. List the factors involved in a successful client consultation.

4. Demonstrate the safe and proper use of the various tools of haircutting.

5. Demonstrate mastery of the four basic haircuts.

6. Demonstrate mastery of other haircutting techniques.

essential **haircutting**

I really want to specialize in hair design, so why is it so important for me to master the art of haircutting?

Haircutting is a technique that requires many hours of practice and a vivid imagination. It is an extremely important skill that must be mastered because the cut serves as the basis for every hairstyle. It may not be done as frequently as a shampoo or style, but it is certainly done more frequently than chemical services. If you want to ensure that the style you provide your clients is attractive and will look good even when they style their own hair, you must deliver a quality haircut. The way to accomplish this is with frequent practice, repetitive exercises, timed procedures, and a strong desire to become an accomplished haircutter.

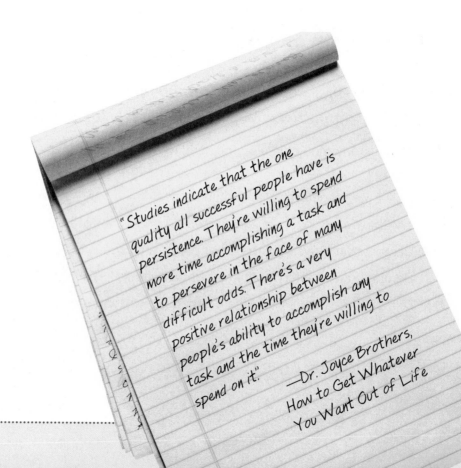

"Studies indicate that the one quality all successful people have is persistence. They're willing to spend more time accomplishing a task and to persevere in the face of many difficult odds. There's a very positive relationship between people's ability to accomplish any task and the time they're willing to spend on it."

—Dr. Joyce Brothers,
How to Get Whatever
You Want Out of Life

essential concepts

What are the most important techniques and procedures I should learn to become a good haircutter?

Haircutting is actually more than just reducing length and bulk from the hair. It begins with using quality tools, and there are many to aid you in achieving a dynamic haircut. You will want to practice techniques with shears, razors, clippers, thinning shears, and all the ancillary tools such as combs and brushes. You will want to work with all these tools until you have complete control and can handle them with ease. You will also need to become familiar with all the terms used in haircutting. It is important to remember that terminology in our industry constantly changes. Don't let yourself get sidetracked because a particular instructor or book calls a specific cut one thing and another calls it something else. It's the end result that matters, not what the technique, procedure, or style is named.

Your instructor will take you through steps of sectioning for various types of cuts. You will find that proper sectioning is extremely important, especially until you have learned to manage and control larger amounts of hair. You will learn about angles and elevations and how to combine them to create a wide variety of hairstyles. It is highly recommended that you style every haircut you complete while learning. This allows you to see the results of your efforts. If, for example, you are unable to achieve the desired style after the cut, it may be because you haven't yet mastered that particular haircut. Just remember that no one performs a perfect haircut the first time. It takes practice and commitment—so don't give up.

essential
experience
1

Identify the Tools

Using the artwork below, label each tool using the following terms (some terms may be used more than once).

back	haircutting shears	pivot screw	tail comb
barber comb	handle	point	tang
blade	head	shank	thinning shears
edge	heel	shoulder	thumb grip
finger grip	moving blade	still blade	wide-tooth comb
finger brace	pivot	styling comb	

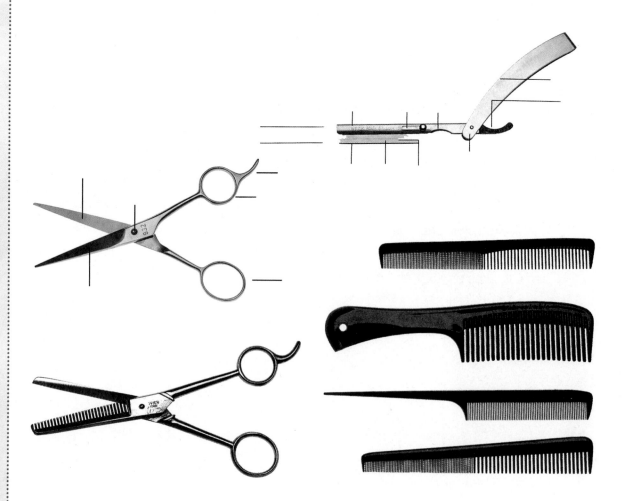

essential 2 experience

Windowpaning is the process of transferring key elements, points, or steps in a lesson into visual images that are hand sketched into the squares or "panes" of a matrix. Let your mind think in pictures and sketch the essential concepts printed in each of the following windowpanes. Don't be concerned with your artistic ability. Use lines and stick figures to depict each concept.

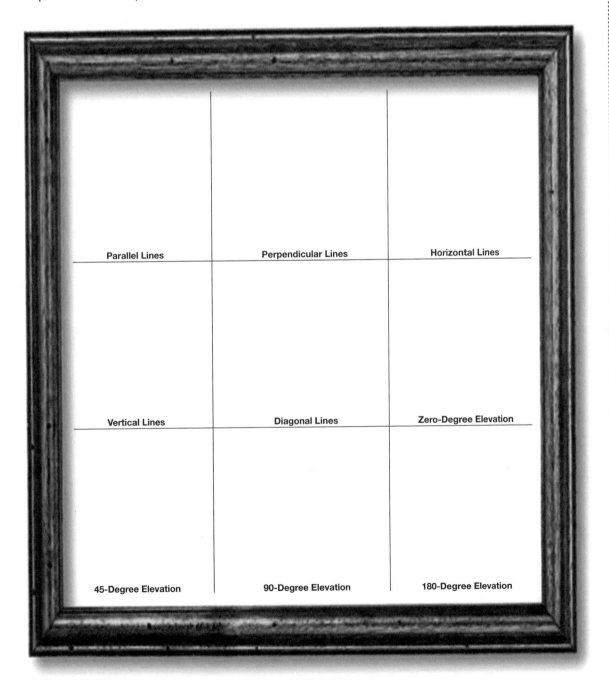

Parallel Lines	Perpendicular Lines	Horizontal Lines
Vertical Lines	Diagonal Lines	Zero-Degree Elevation
45-Degree Elevation	90-Degree Elevation	180-Degree Elevation

essential
3 experience

Match each of the following essential terms with its definition.

_____ Beveled cut

_____ Blunt cut

_____ Elevation

_____ Graduated

_____ Guide

_____ Layering

_____ Notching or pointing

_____ Parting

_____ Sections

_____ Tension

_____ Weight line

_____ Shears

_____ Thinning shears

_____ Razor

_____ Clippers

_____ Edgers

_____ Parallel lines

_____ Perpendicular lines

_____ Horizontal lines

_____ Vertical lines

_____ Diagonal lines

1. Lines that are between horizontal and vertical.
2. Two lines that intersect at a 90-degree angle.
3. Used to remove superfluous hair and to create clean lines around the perimeter of a short taper.
4. Used to create very short tapers quickly.
5. Usually used to cut a blunt straight line. Can be used to thin hair by slithering.
6. Lines that are parallel to the floor; used in low elevation haircuts.
7. Two or more lines that do not meet in space.
8. Used to remove bulk from the hair.
9. Used to cut hair with a softer edge than shears.
10. Holding the shears at an angle other than 90 degrees to the hair strand.
11. Cutting with the points of the shears to create texture in the hair ends.
12. Shape with a stacked area around the exterior that is cut at low-to-medium elevations.
13. Graduated effect achieved by cutting the hair with elevation or overdirection.
14. Section of hair that determines the length the hair will be cut.
15. Level at which a blunt cut falls; where the ends of the hair hang together.
16. Used for control when cutting; also called subsection.
17. How tightly the hair is pulled before cutting.
18. Lines that are perpendicular to the floor.
19. Cutting the hair straight across the strand. All hair hangs to one level, forming a weight line.
20. Divisions of the hair made before cutting.
21. Angle at which the hair is held away from the head for cutting.

essential experience
4

Windowpaning is the process of transferring key elements, points, or steps in a lesson into visual images that are hand sketched into the squares or "panes" of a matrix. Let your mind think in pictures and sketch the essential concepts printed in each of the following windowpanes. Don't be concerned with your artistic ability. Use lines and stick figures to depict each concept.

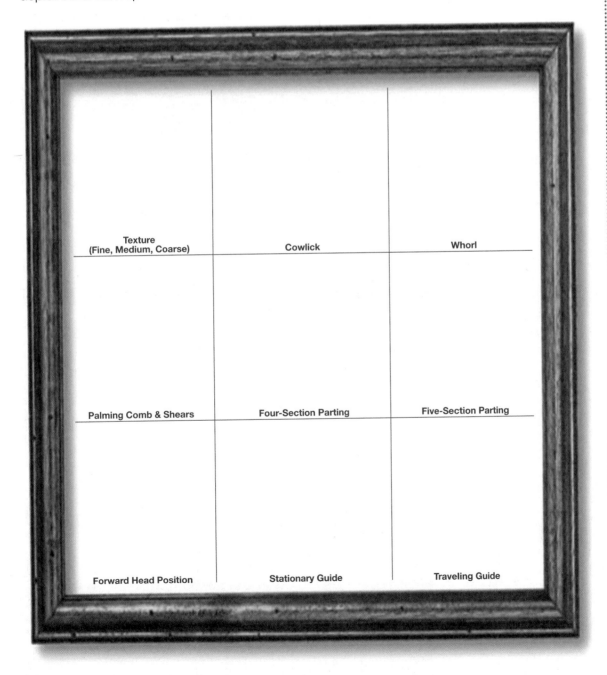

Texture (Fine, Medium, Coarse)	Cowlick	Whorl
Palming Comb & Shears	Four-Section Parting	Five-Section Parting
Forward Head Position	Stationary Guide	Traveling Guide

essential
5 experience

As a professional stylist you will have numerous clients who bring in photographs because they want to achieve the same or similar look. Therefore, learning how to evaluate a style and determine how it was achieved will be of great benefit to you. With that in mind, look through various magazines and select three particular cuts that appeal to you. Paste them on the chart below in the left column. In the right column, diagram and/or explain the techniques, angles, and elevations you would use to create this particular haircut and style.

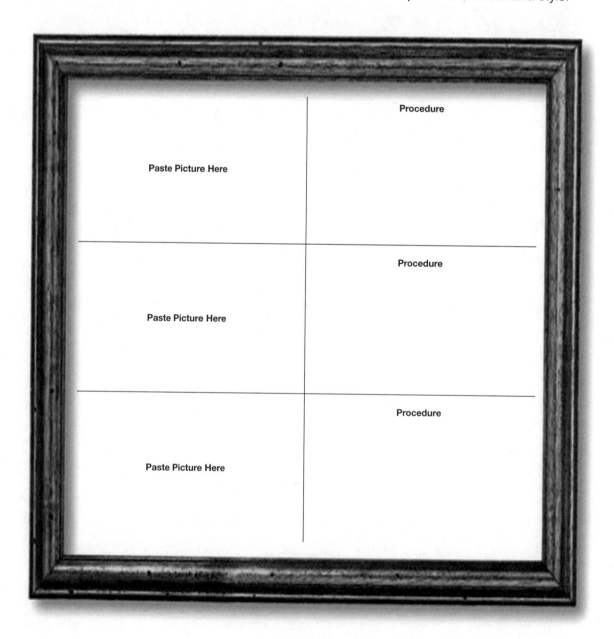

	Procedure
Paste Picture Here	
Paste Picture Here	**Procedure**
Paste Picture Here	**Procedure**

essential experience 6

Word Scramble

Scramble	Correct Word
ntlub uct	_ _ _ _ _ _ _ _ _ *Clue:* Cut straight across
adterudga	_ _ _ _ _ _ _ _ _ *Clue:* A wedge or stack
eeevrsr	_ _ _ _ _ _ _ *Clue:* 180-degree elevation
egrynial	_ _ _ _ _ _ _ _ *Clue:* Each subsection slightly shorter than guide
iseontcs	_ _ _ _ _ _ _ _ *Clue:* Divisions in hair before cutting
ladnioag	_ _ _ _ _ _ _ _ *Clue:* Between horizontal and vertical
lenaigvrt	_ _ _ _ _ _ _ _ _ *Clue:* Moving
liavctre	_ _ _ _ _ _ _ _ *Clue:* Perpendicular to the floor
diew hotot	_ _ _ _ _ _ _ _ _ *Clue:* Comb used to create softer edge when cutting with shears
sderge	_ _ _ _ _ _ *Clue:* Removes superfluous hair
utsenoicsb	_ _ _ _ _ _ _ _ _ _ *Clue:* Partings
hrlwo	_ _ _ _ _ *Clue:* Requires extra length
zroar	_ _ _ _ _ *Clue:* Cuts hair with softer edge

essential experience

7

Word Search

After determining the correct words from the clues provided, locate the words in the word search puzzle.

Word	Clue
_____	Used for close tapers
_____	Holding the shears at an angle other than 90 degrees to the hair strand
_____	A cut that is short on the bottom and long on the top
_____	Cheaters
_____	Found in the hairline or the interior of the hair
_____	Slithering
_____	The angle at which the hair is held away from the head
_____	Section of hair that determines the length
_____	90-degree haircut
_____	Lines that are parallel to the floor

```
B A R B E R C O M B M G L Q T B
I N S X W E C H D Q V M S W L I
H K E D L F B C H F M W N E D G
M Q I D R Q U P I G Y O N W P T
Y E A W I A B S F R I D Q C F B
N M Q S S U U Q Q T E E M N U G
O R N X P X G G A D J C H R J N
I I X T C S Q V H Q V A O J X I
T Q H B C Y E T S T L T X I O T
A H D W P L H S P K G V W T K A
V M C E E T R X I G C N P D K L
E G L H G A N K Y V B I E X Y I
L V G E W E N J U H V R L L Y F
E I A F D J J I I S H S E W C F
H H O R I Z O N T A L Z F F O E
B E V E L E D C U T W B X I C C
```

essential experience

8

In your own words, explain the purpose of the following procedures.

Checking a Haircut

Learning to check your own haircuts before requesting assistance from an instructor will save you and your client wasted time.

_____

_____

_____

_____

_____

Slide Cutting

You will find this technique extremely beneficial in removing length or for texturizing to create an attractive style for your clients.

_____

_____

_____

_____

_____

Scissors-over-Comb Technique

You'll find this technique especially beneficial in giving short haircuts to both men and women!

_____

_____

_____

_____

essential
9 experience

Word Search

After determining the correct words from the clues provided, locate the words in the word search puzzle.

Word	Clue
_____	Traveling
_____	Also known as pointing
_____	Lines that never meet in space
_____	Subsections
_____	A popular barbering technique
_____	Used to cut a blunt straight line across the hair
_____	Stable
_____	How tightly the hair is pulled when cutting
_____	Removing bulk without removing length
_____	Level at which the blunt cut falls

```
G  E  M  N  F  P  Y  L  H  D  G  W  B  C  S  T
I  N  D  O  X  H  H  K  Q  I  S  Q  V  C  E  R
J  U  I  I  V  R  M  Q  T  A  L  R  I  N  S  E
R  E  X  T  U  I  Y  F  A  A  O  S  S  X  F  I
L  P  A  M  R  G  N  R  F  Y  S  I  M  Z  V  Z
O  S  X  V  J  A  Y  G  K  O  O  L  S  A  B  S
G  Z  I  P  U  X  P  R  R  N  B  N  S  J  C  G
N  C  W  F  L  N  N  O  A  V  I  U  N  G  A  N
I  Q  B  W  U  Y  V  P  G  N  I  O  G  B  I  I
T  S  O  G  T  E  A  Y  A  N  O  R  V  S  Y  N
N  L  U  F  R  R  F  B  I  Y  I  I  Z  F  S  N
I  V  T  C  A  G  Q  U  G  C  F  H  T  B  I  I
O  G  O  L  D  S  G  H  W  P  Z  Q  C  A  A  H
P  M  L  K  Y  N  A  J  X  T  F  W  W  T  T  T
B  E  W  Z  T  O  I  E  H  F  R  P  J  S  O  S
L  W  E  I  G  H  T  L  I  N  E  H  S  Q  B  N
```

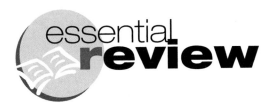

essential review

Complete the following review of Chapter 11, "Haircutting," by circling the correct answer to each question.

1. Cutting the hair straight across the strand is a/an _____ cut.

a) elevation   b) blunt

c) graduated   d) beveled

2. A cut that has a stacked area around the exterior and is cut at low-to-medium elevations is a/an _____ cut.

a) elevation   b) blunt

c) graduated   d) beveled

3. Cutting with the points of the shears to create texture is known as _____ .

a) layering   b) undercutting

c) elevation   d) notching

4. Subdivisions of a section used for control when cutting, are known as

_____ .

a) parting   b) guides

c) sections   d) tension

5. If the hair is cut partially wet and partially dry, the results will be _____ .

a) even   b) perfect

c) uneven   d) curly

6. The tool used to create clean lines around the perimeter of a short taper is the

_____ .

a) clippers   b) edgers

c) razor   d) shears

7. A tool used to cut blunt straight lines is called the _____ .

a) clippers   b) edgers

c) razor   d) shears

8. The tool used to cut hair with a softer edge is know as the _____ .

a) clippers   b) edgers

c) razor   d) shears

9. The comb used for close tapers in the nape and sides is the _____ comb.

a) styling   b) barber

c) wide-tooth   d) tail

essential review *continued*

10. The comb used to create a softer edge when cutting with the shears is the
_____ comb.

    a) styling   b) barber

    c) wide-tooth   d) tail

11. _____ points are points on the head that mark where the surface of the head
changes or the behavior of the hair changes, such as the ears, jawline, occipital bone, or
apex.

    a) parietal   b) crown

    c) elevation   d) reference

12. Two or more lines that do not meet in space are _____ lines.

    a) parallel   b) perpendicular

    c) diagonal   d) vertical

13. Lines that are perpendicular to the floor are _____ lines.

    a) parallel   b) perpendicular

    c) diagonal   d) vertical

14. Two lines that intersect at a 90-degree angle are _____ lines.

    a) parallel   b) perpendicular

    c) diagonal   d) vertical

15. Lines that are used for blending and special design haircuts are _____ lines.

    a) parallel   b) perpendicular

    c) diagonal   d) vertical

16. A stable guide that does not move is also known as a _____ guide.

    a) moving   b) traveling

    c) stationary   d) mobile

17. A 90-degree haircut is also known as a _____-elevation cut.

    a) low   b) high

    c) reverse   d) blended

18. A 180-degree haircut is also known as a _____ .

    a) low-elevation cut   b) combined-elevation cut

    c) long layered haircut   d) blended-elevation cut

19. A zero-degree haircut is also known as a _____-elevation cut.

    a) low   b) high

    c) reverse   d) blended

essential review *continued*

20. A barbering technique that has become popular with cosmetologists is the
_____-over-comb method.

a) clipper   b) razor

c) trimmer   d) shears

21. A/an _____ is a thin continuous mark used as a guide.

a) angle   b) line

c) elevation   d) section

22. A method of cutting or thinning the hair using razor-sharp shears is called
_____ cutting.

a) point   b) slide

c) notching   d) razor

23. The process of thinning with shears is known as _____ .

a) effilating   b) shaving

c) sliding   d) trimming

24. _____ guides are used mostly in blunt (one-length) haircuts or when using
overdirection to create a length or weight increase in a haircut.

a) traveling   b) movable

c) stationary   d) portable

25. _____ is used mostly in graduated and layered haircuts, and in those
situations where a length increase in the design is desired.

a) effilating   b) trimming

c) elevating   d) overdirection

essential discoveries and accomplishments

In the space below, jot some notes about what concepts of this chapter were hardest for you to understand or remember. Imagine finding yourself suddenly in the role of "teacher" and consider what you would tell your "students" about these difficult concepts.

Share your *Essential Discoveries* with some of the other students in your class and ask if they are helpful to them. You may want to revise your notes based on good ideas shared by your peers. Under "Accomplishments," list at least three things you have accomplished since your last entry that relate to your career goals.

Discoveries:

_____

_____

_____

_____

_____

Accomplishments:

_____

_____

_____

_____

_____

chapter 12

Hairstyling

essential **objectives**

After studying this chapter and completing the Essential Companion *components, you should be able to:*

1. Explain the importance of learning the various wet hairstyling techniques.

2. Demonstrate the techniques of finger waving, pin curls, roller setting, and hair wrapping.

3. Demonstrate two basic techniques of styling long hair.

4. Demonstrate mastery of various blow-dry styling techniques.

5. Demonstrate the proper use of thermal irons.

6. Demonstrate the thermal iron manipulations and explain how they are used.

7. Describe the three types of hair pressing.

8. Demonstrate the procedures involved in soft pressing and hard pressing.

9. List the safety precautions that must be observed in thermal styling and hair pressing.

essential wet hairstyling

What roles will wet hairstyling, thermal hairstyling, and hair pressing play in my success as a cosmetologist?

Hairstyles, like fashions, are cyclical. Just as you've seen the bell-bottom pants of the late 1960s come into fashion again, hairstyles such as those that were popular in the 1920s surface from time to time in our society. History has shown that all societies have cut and arranged hair to modify its natural state. The pages of our history books depict great diversity from era to era. They show the blonde wigs of Roman matrons, the gray wigs of English barristers, and the black wigs of the Japanese geisha. We also see the sleek, waved look worn by the flappers in the 1920s and the trend toward informality and individualism in the twenty-first century.

Recent surveys of today's modern salons indicate that the new stylists joining their teams must be skilled in many styling techniques, including thermal styling and curling. History shows us that thermal or heat techniques have been used for centuries to create certain looks. The heat from the sun was used to speed up the processing of hair lighteners, permanent waves, and haircolor. Hair was wrapped around reeds and sticks and sun-dried for certain looks. Fortunately, the tools and implements have improved drastically since those primitive times.

Marcel Grateau developed the thermal iron technique in 1875, which is still called marcel waving today. The use of blow drying and curling irons became really popular in the late 1960s with the first "bob" cut. These techniques have become increasingly popular into the twenty-first century as more women have entered the business world where time is so critical. These techniques are used for what are called "quick services" in the salon. However, the same care must be taken with these techniques as with wet hairstyling.

essential wet hairstyling *continued*

Hair pressing is both a popular and profitable service that is used in many of today's professional establishments. Extremely curly hair comes in many colors, textures, and ethnicity. We have all heard the expression, "The grass looks greener on the other side of the fence." We human beings always seem to want something that we don't have. If we have straight hair, we want it to be curly; so we seek out chemical texture services to add curl to our hair. If we have naturally curly hair, we want it to be straight; so we seek out either pressing or chemical services to remove the curl. All those client desires contribute to your success as a professional cosmetologist.

Once you become a professional cosmetologist, you will hold your license or certification for many years (hopefully several decades). You must be prepared to address your client's desires and needs regardless of the prevailing styles of the times. Therefore, it is essential that you learn the basics of hairstyling in order to be proficient in providing the client's desired style.

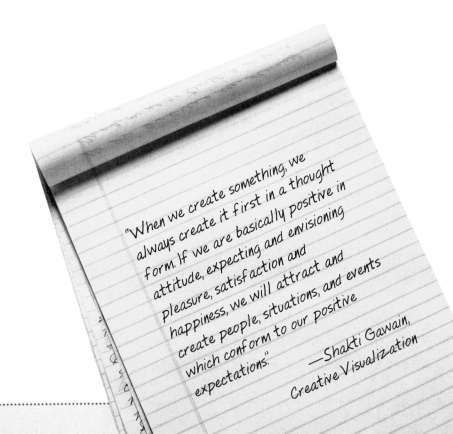

"When we create something, we always create it first in a thought form. If we are basically positive in attitude, expecting and envisioning pleasure, satisfaction and happiness, we will attract and create people, situations, and events which conform to our positive expectations."

—Shakti Gawain, *Creative Visualization*

essential wet hairstyling concepts

What are the most important elements in hairstyling that I need to know?

Hairstyling is an art form; hair is the medium and you are the artist. Hairstyling results from a detailed set of principles, elements, tools, and implements. You will need to master the use of the tools and implements used in hairstyling as well as how to properly prepare the hair for the styling service. You will become familiar with a variety of styling aids which do just that—aid you in creating the desired look or style. For example, you will learn that finger waving is the art of shaping and directing the hair into alternate parallel waves with well-defined ridges using the fingers, combs, and waving lotion.

You will learn how the concept of waves evolves into the concept of curls, including pin curls and roller curls. There are a variety of techniques for creating pin curls and roller sets which will allow you to work your magic as an artist in your medium of hair. You will also master several brushing and combing techniques so that you can give a finished look to the style you have designed.

In addition, thermal styling is the art of drying, waving, and curling hair by means of heat, using special manipulative techniques. It includes drying and styling the hair, curling or waving the hair, and straightening the hair. Each piece of equipment used in thermal styling is designed for a specific styling technique. The essential techniques that you must master are the use of the blow-dryer and the curling iron. You will need to know how each piece of equipment functions and how to create a variety of looks with each.

You will also need to learn about the three types of hair-pressing techniques: the soft press, the medium press, and the hard press. It is essential that you understand which type of press is used on which type of hair. Of course, you will also need to master each of the techniques. Learning about special problems with pressing and fine-tuning all the safety measures that must be followed will also contribute to your success.

essential experience 1

Mind Map of Wet Hairstyling

Mind mapping simply creates a free-flowing outline of material or information with the key point being located in the center. The key point of this mind map is Wet Hairstyling. Diagram the different tools, implements, and elements or categories of wet hairstyling. Use terms, pictures, and symbols as desired. Using color will increase the mind's retention and memory of the material. Keep your mind open and uncluttered, and don't worry about where a line or word should go; the organization of the map will usually take care of itself.

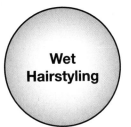

essential
2experience

Windowpane—Pin Curls

Windowpaning is the process of transferring key elements, points, or steps in a lesson into visual images that are hand sketched into the squares or "panes" of a matrix. Let your mind think in pictures and sketch the essential concepts printed in each of the following windowpanes. Don't be concerned with your artistic ability. Use lines and stick figures to depict the concepts indicated.

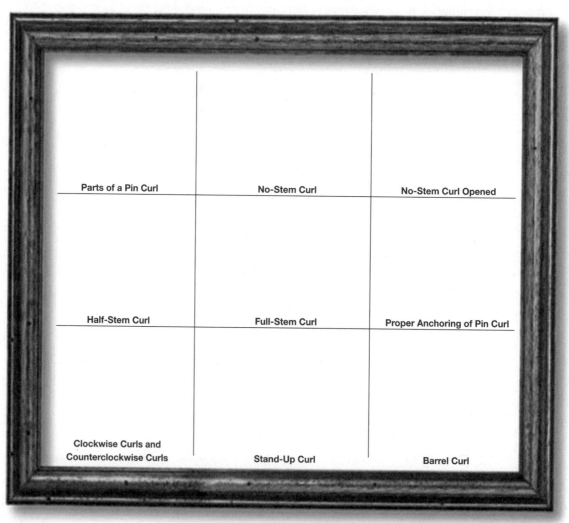

Parts of a Pin Curl	No-Stem Curl	No-Stem Curl Opened
Half-Stem Curl	Full-Stem Curl	Proper Anchoring of Pin Curl
Clockwise Curls and Counterclockwise Curls	Stand-Up Curl	Barrel Curl

Follow-up Activity: Perform each of the following curls or movements on a mannequin for a grade from your instructor.

____ No-Stem Curl   ____ Stand-Up Curl   ____ Full-Stem Curl

____ Clockwise Curl   ____ Half-Stem Curl   ____ Barrel Curl

essential
3experience

Pin Curl Shaping and Bases

Match the following essential terms with their identifying phrase or definition.

_____ Skip waves

_____ No-stem curl

_____ Shaping

_____ Ridge curls

_____ Spiral curls

_____ Carved curls

_____ Closed center
curls

_____ Rectangular base

_____ Triangular base

_____ Arc base

_____ Square base

_____ Ribboning

1. Pin curls sliced from a shaping and formed without lifting the hair from the head.

2. Two rows of ridge curls, usually on the side of the head.

3. Recommended along the front or facial hairline to avoid breaks or splits in the finished style.

4. Pin curl placed directly on the base of the curl that produces a tight, firm, long-lasting curl.

5. Used for even construction suitable for curly hairstyles without much volume or lift.

6. Also known as the half-moon or C-shape base.

7. Recommended at front hairline for a smooth upsweep effect.

8. Section of hair molded in a circular motion.

9. Pin curls that produce waves that get smaller in size toward the end.

10. Pin curls placed behind or below a ridge to form a wave.

11. Forcing the strand through the comb while applying pressure with the thumb on the back of the comb to create tension.

12. Method of curling hair by winding strand around the rod.

essential
4 experience

Windowpane—Roller Placement

Windowpaning is the process of transferring key elements, points, or steps in a lesson into visual images that are hand sketched into the squares or "panes" of a matrix. Let your mind think in pictures and sketch the essential concepts printed in each of the following windowpanes. Don't be concerned with your artistic ability. Use lines and stick figures to depict the concepts indicated.

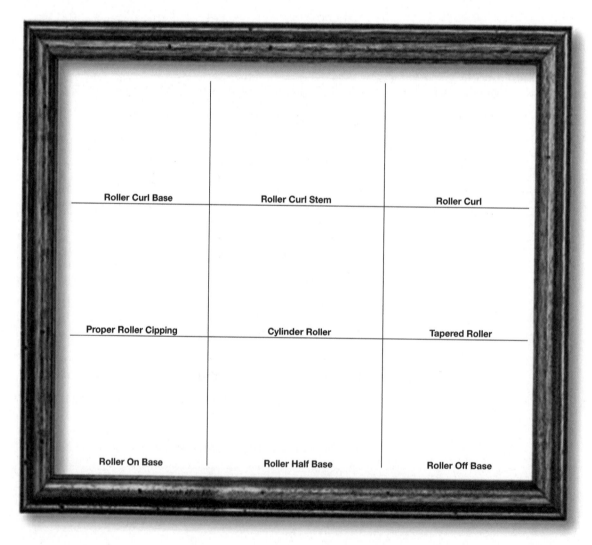

Roller Curl Base	Roller Curl Stem	Roller Curl
Proper Roller Cipping	Cylinder Roller	Tapered Roller
Roller On Base	Roller Half Base	Roller Off Base

essential
experience
5

Word Search

After identifying the appropriate word from the clues listed below, locate the word in the following word search puzzle.

_____ Also called ruffing

_____ Pin curls with large openings; fastened to the head in a standing position on a rectangular base

_____ Pin curls sliced from a shaping and formed without lifting the hair from the head

_____ Nozzle attachment that directs the air flow

_____ Blow-dryer attachment that causes air to flow more softly

_____ Technique of passing a hot curling iron through the hair before performing a hard press

_____ Produces a strong curl with full volume

_____ Removes 100 percent of the curl by applying the pressing comb twice on each side of the hair

_____ Curl placed directly on its base

_____ Forcing hair between the thumb and back of the comb to create tension

_____ Pin curls placed immediately behind or below a ridge to form a wave

_____ Round, solid prong of a thermal iron

_____ Part of thermal irons in which the rod rests when irons are closed

_____ Two rows of ridge curls, usually on the side of the head

_____ Method of curling the hair by winding a strand around the rod

_____ Also called cascade curls

_____ Section of pin curl between the base and first arc

_____ Hairstyle arranged up and off the shoulders

_____ Type of gel that makes hair pliable for finger waving

```
S  L  R  U  C  L  E  R  R  A  B  S  T  G  M
L  R  U  C  L  A  R  I  P  S  B  G  N  N  K
R  E  S  N  O  I  T  O  L  G  N  I  V  A  W
U  S  L  D  S  M  T  R  G  I  H  U  Q  K  Q
C  U  R  W  O  I  O  O  N  S  S  S  U  M  X
P  F  U  S  M  U  O  O  U  N  S  W  S  M  B
U  F  C  B  L  P  B  R  S  H  E  L  L  E  U
-  I  D  M  D  B  B  L  Q  W  R  A  F  T  R
D  D  E  H  I  -  J  D  E  U  P  D  O  S  H
N  O  V  R  K  V  X  Y  C  P  D  F  E  -  T
A  X  R  C  O  N  C  E  N  T  R  A  T  O  R
T  L  A  E  P  H  G  N  I  C  A  E  R  N  N
S  B  C  J  J  D  F  O  K  J  H  D  S  H  B
Z  R  S  K  I  P  W  A  V  E  S  Z  H  S  Q
I  T  I  R  E  S  A  R  -  L  L  U  E  S  T
```

essential
experience
6

Thermal Irons

Identify the essential parts of the conventional thermal or marcel iron and the electric thermal iron below. Parts include: rod, shell, rod handle, shell handle, and swivel.

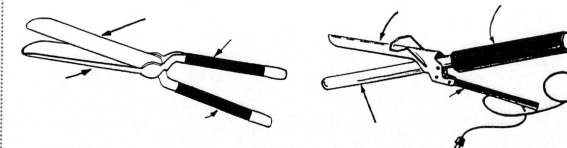

Conventional thermal (marcel) iron   **Electric thermal iron**

After identifying the essential parts of the irons, please state in your own words the procedure for testing the heat of a thermal iron.

_____

_____

_____

_____

_____

essential experience
7

Iron Manipulations

Using a cold thermal iron, a mannequin, and other required implements, practice the textbook exercises for manipulating thermal irons.

Exercise 1:   Since it is important to develop a smooth rotating movement, practice turning the irons while opening and closing them at regular intervals. Practice rotating the irons downward toward you and upward away from you.

Exercise 2:   Practice releasing the hair by opening and closing the irons in a quick, clicking movement.

Exercise 3:   Practice guiding the hair strand into the center of the curl as you rotate the irons. This exercise will ensure that the end of the strand is firmly in the center of the curl.

Exercise 4:   Practice removing the curl from the irons by drawing the comb to the left and the rod to the right. Use the comb to protect the scalp from burns.

After completing the exercises, please explain any difficulties you may have had with the exercises in the space below. Discuss these difficulties with your instructor.

essential
experience
8

Safety Precautions

In the space provided, explain why the following safety precautions are necessary when thermal waving and/or curling.

1. Irons should not be overheated.

_____

2. The temperature of the irons must be tested before applying to hair.

_____

3. Irons should be handled carefully.

_____

4. Irons should be placed in a safe place to cool.

_____

5. Handles should not be placed too close to the heater when heating the irons.

_____

6. Irons should be properly balanced when placed in the heater.

_____

7. Celluloid combs or metal combs cannot be used.

_____

8. Combs with broken teeth must not be used.

_____

9. Comb must be placed between scalp and thermal iron when curling or waving.

_____

10. Hair ends must not be allowed to protrude over the irons.

_____

11. Thermal irons are generally not used on chemically straightened hair.

_____

12. A first aid kit must be readily available.

_____

essential
experience

Thermal Curling Preparation

Please list the five general steps used in preparing for an electric or stove-heated thermal curling iron procedure. Bear in mind that these methods may be changed by your instructor.

1. _____

   _____

   _____

2. _____

   _____

   _____

3. _____

   _____

   _____

4. _____

   _____

   _____

5. _____

   _____

   _____

essential
experience
10

Windowpaning—Thermal Curling

Windowpaning is the process of transferring key elements, points, or steps in a lesson into visual images that are hand sketched into the squares or "panes" of a matrix. Let your mind think in pictures and sketch the essential concepts printed in each of the following windowpanes. Don't be concerned with your artistic ability. Use lines and stick figures to depict the concepts requested.

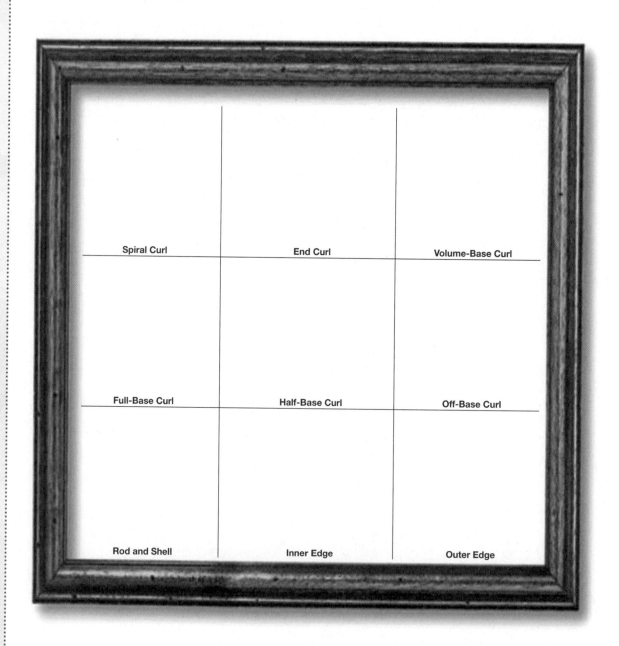

Spiral Curl	End Curl	Volume-Base Curl
Full-Base Curl	Half-Base Curl	Off-Base Curl
Rod and Shell	Inner Edge	Outer Edge

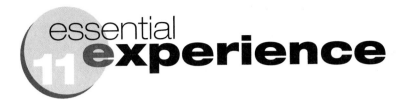

essential experience 11

Thermal Waving with Conventional Thermal Irons

List below the equipment, implements, and materials used in thermal waving with a conventional thermal (marcel) iron.

_____

_____

ANSWER:

In your own words, list the basic procedural steps that can be used to create a style with a conventional thermal (marcel) iron for a left-going wave.

1. _____

_____

_____

_____

2. _____

_____

_____

_____

3. _____

_____

_____

_____

4. _____

_____

_____

_____

5. _____

_____

_____

_____

6. _____

_____

_____

_____

7. _____

_____

_____

_____

8. _____

_____

_____

_____

9. _____

_____

_____

_____

10. _____

_____

_____

_____

11. _____

_____

_____

_____

12. _____

_____

_____

_____

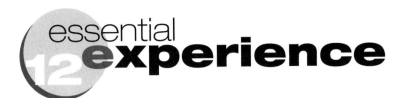

Types of Hair Pressing

In your own words and in the space provided, explain what is meant by each type of pressing technique and how each is accomplished.

SOFT PRESS: _____

_____

MEDIUM PRESS: _____

_____

_____

HARD PRESS: _____

_____

_____

essential
13experience

Product Knowledge

Research a variety of pressing oils or creams available in your school and found at local supply stores. Use the chart below to track your findings.

Product Name	Key Ingredients	Purpose	Benefits	Directions for Use

essential
14 experience

Hair and Scalp Analysis

List the eight points that should be thoroughly covered in the hair and scalp analysis before proceeding with a hair pressing service.

1. _____

2. _____

3. _____

4. _____

5. _____

6. _____

7. _____

8. _____

List at least five reminders and hints on soft pressing.

1. _____
   _____

2. _____
   _____

3. _____
   _____

4. _____
   _____

5. _____
   _____

6. _____
   _____

7. _____
   _____

essential
15 experience

Jeopardy

As in the game of *Jeopardy,* write questions that would be correctly answered as follows:

Hair Pressing for $100

1. To temporarily straighten extremely curly or unruly hair

_____

2. A series of conditioning treatments

_____

_____

3. Soft, medium, hard

_____

Hair Pressing for $200

1. Double press

_____

2. Breakage

_____

3. Medium hair

_____

Hair Pressing for $300

1. Scalp abrasions, contagious scalp condition, scalp injury, chemically treated hair

_____

2. Wiry, curly hair

_____

3. Regular and electric

_____

Hair Pressing for $400

1. Carbon

_____

2. Apply less pressure to the hair near the ends

_____

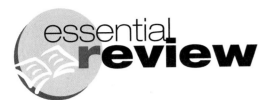
essential **review**

Using the following words, fill in the blanks below to form a thorough review of Chapter 12, "Hairstyling." Words or terms may be used more than once or not at all.

anchored	decrease	invisible	ridge
arc	direction	no	rollers
back combing	drying	oblong	ruffing
barrel	finger waving	off	shallow
base	flattering	on	silicone shiners
C-shaped	full	pinching	smooth
carved	gel	pin curls	square
circle	karaya	pins	stand-up
circular	finishing	pliable	stem
clockwise	full	pomade	tapered
counterclockwise	hairpins	pushing	tension
curls	horizontal	rectangular	vertical
cylinder	indentation	ribboning	visible

1. No matter what the client says during a client consultation, what he or she really wants is a style that is _____ and easy to maintain.

2. Open center curls produce even, _____ waves and uniform curls.

3. In _____ finger waving, ridges are parallel around the head.

4. One complete turn around the roller will create a _____ curl.

5. The art of shaping and directing the hair into alternate parallel waves and designs is _____ .

6. The three parts of a pin curl are the _____, _____, and _____ .

7. The finished result will be determined by the _____ you place the stem of the curl.

8. Curls formed in the opposite direction of the movement of the hands of a clock are known as _____ .

9. Forcing a strand of hair through a comb while applying pressure with the thumb on the back of the comb to create tension is called _____ .

essential review *continued*

10. _____ are used to create many of the same effects as stand-up pin curls.

11. Two and a half turns around the roller will create _____.

12. Curls formed in the same direction as the movement of the hands of a clock are known as _____.

13. The most commonly shaped base you will use is the _____ base.

14. Cascade or _____ curls are used to create height.

15. For the least volume, the roller sits _____ base.

16. Tools and implements required in wet hairstyling include rollers, clips, combs, brushes, and _____.

17. Waving lotion makes the hair _____ and keeps it in place during the finger waving procedure.

18. A _____ curl allows for the greatest mobility.

19. Waving lotion is applied to one side of the head at a time to prevent _____.

20. _____ provide the bases for patterns, lines, waves, curls, and rolls that you can use to create hairstyles.

21. Closed center curls produce waves that _____ in size.

22. Do not try to increase the height or depth of a ridge by _____ or _____ with fingers.

23. Waving lotion is made from _____ gum.

24. A loose roller will lose its _____ and result in a weak set.

25. Secure finger waves with _____ if needed.

26. In _____ finger waving, ridges run up and down the head.

27. Back brushing is also known as _____.

28. _____ is a firm-bodied and usually clear or transparent product that comes in a tube or bottle and has a strong hold.

29. To ensure that the curl holds firmly, it should be _____ correctly.

30. Pin curls recommended at the side front hairline for smooth upsweep effect are _____ bases.

31. Pin curls sliced from a shaping without lifting hair from the head are referred to as _____ curls.

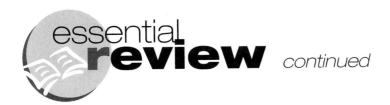

essential **review** *continued*

32. For full volume, the roller sits _____ base.

33. Large stand-up pin curls on a rectangular base with large center openings are known as _____ curls.

34. Teasing, ratting, matting, or French lacing are also known as _____.

35. _____ or wax add considerable weight to the hair by causing strands to join together.

36. A _____ stem curl produces a tight, firm, long lasting curl.

37. _____ add gloss and sheen to the hair while creating textural definition.

38. A _____ curl is a wave behind the ridge.

39. The most widely used hairstyling product is hair spray or _____ spray.

Please complete the following multiple choice questions by circling the correct answer.

40. When blow-drying, determine the size of the brush to be used by the desired style and _____ of the hair.

    a) elasticity   b) texture

    c) length   d) porosity

41. The styling parts of the thermal iron are the rod and the _____.

    a) groove   b) handle

    c) shell   d) clamp

42. The temperature of the heated thermal iron is tested on _____.

    a) wax paper   b) a hair strand

    c) a damp cloth   d) tissue paper

43. Curling with two loops is also known as _____ curling.

    a) end   b) spiral

    c) figure eight   d) half-base

44. The technique of waving and curling the hair known as marcel waving is also called _____.

    a) blow-drying   b) thermal waving

    c) heat rolling   d) finger waving

45. Combs for thermal curling should be made of _____.

    a) celluloid   b) hard rubber

    c) plastic   d) soft rubber

46. To give a finished appearance to hair ends, use _____ curls.

    a) figure eight   b) loop

    c) figure six   d) end

47. For successful blow-dry styling, the air should be directed from the scalp to the

    _____ .

    a) floor   b) ceiling

    c) face   d) ends

48. When the blow-dry style is complete, the scalp must be _____ .

    a) oily   b) moist

    c) damp   d) dry

49. Overheated irons are often ruined because the metal loses its _____ .

    a) color   b) balance

    c) temper   d) strength

50. Electric vaporizing irons should not be used on pressed hair because they cause the hair

    to _____ .

    a) break   b) dry

    c) straighten   d) revert

51. _____ hair withstands less heat in a thermal styling service than normal

    hair.

    a) lightened   b) healthy

    c) coarse   d) curly

52. A conventional thermal iron is _____ heated.

    a) electric   b) self

    c) coal   d) stove

53. _____ hair, as a rule, can tolerate more heat than fine hair.

    a) red   b) coarse

    c) oily   d) short

54. Spiral curls are hanging curls that are suitable for _____ hairstyles.

    a) short   b) clipped

    c) long   d) straight

55. Until dexterity is achieved and ease of manipulation is mastered, it is best to practice with

    _____ irons.

    a) cold   b) hot

    c) warm   d) rigid

essential review *continued*

56. How long does a hair press last?

    a) a week

    b) till the next haircut

    c) overnight

    d) till the next shampoo

57. The types of hair pressing are soft, medium, and _____ .

    a) light

    b) hard

    c) extreme

    d) heavy

58. The temperature of the pressing comb and the amount of pressure used is adjusted based on the _____ of the hair.

    a) texture

    b) length

    c) style

    d) cleanliness

59. Which type of hair requires the most pressure and heat?

    a) fine

    b) medium

    c) normal

    d) wiry

60. Which type of hair requires less pressure and heat than any other type?

    a) fine

    b) medium

    c) coarse

    d) wiry

61. When pressing gray hair, use moderate heat and _____ .

    a) more pressing oil

    b) moderate pressure

    c) less pressure

    d) a larger pressing comb

62. Applying a heated comb twice on each side of the hair is known as a _____ .

    a) regular press

    b) hard press

    c) soft press

    d) comb press

63. Test the temperature of a pressing comb on _____ .

    a) the inner wrist

    b) a terry cloth towel

    c) light paper

    d) dark paper

64. Burnt hair strands _____ .

    a) need extra pressing oil

    b) occur in hard presses

    c) cannot be straightened

    d) cannot be conditioned

65. Using excess heat on gray, tinted, or lightened hair may _____ the hair.

    a) discolor

    b) highlight

    c) strengthen

    d) curl

66. Failure to correct dry and brittle hair can result in hair _____ during hair pressing.

    a) curling

    b) discoloration

    c) strengthening

    d) breakage

essential review *continued*

67. Hair pressing treatments between shampoos are called _____ .

    a) re-presses   b) re-do's

    c) touch-ups   d) soft press

68. Before performing a hair press, the hair should be sectioned into _____ main sections.

    a) 3   b) 4

    c) 5   d) 9

69. Carbon may be removed from the pressing comb by rubbing with _____ .

    a) a wet towel   b) pressing oil

    c) strong alcohol   d) fine steel wool

70. In a hair pressing procedure, the actual pressing or straightening of the hair is accomplished with the comb's _____ .

    a) back rod   b) wide teeth

    c) warm handle   d) narrow tail

71. After cleaning the comb's surface, immerse the comb in a hot _____ solution for about one hour to give the metal a smooth and shiny appearance.

    a) 70 percent alcohol   b) baking soda

    c) soapy water   d) clear ammonia

72. Too frequent hair pressings can cause _____ .

    a) increased strength   b) excessive oiliness

    c) reduced oiliness   d) progressive breakage

73. Pressing combs should be constructed of good-quality stainless steel or _____ .

    a) zinc   b) rubber

    c) brass   d) plastic

74. In pressing coarse hair, more heat is required because it has the greatest _____ .

    a) elasticity   b) length

    c) porosity   d) diameter

75. Handles of pressing combs are usually made of _____ .

    a) wood   b) steel

    c) carbon   d) brass

essential
discoveries and
accomplishments

In the space below, jot some notes about what concepts of this chapter were hardest for you to understand or remember. Imagine finding yourself suddenly in the role of "teacher" and consider what you would tell your "students" about these difficult concepts.

Share your *Essential Discoveries* with some of the other students in your class and ask if they are helpful to them. You may want to revise your notes based on good ideas shared by your peers. Under "Accomplishments," list at least three things you have accomplished since your last entry that relate to your career goals.

Discoveries:

_____

_____

_____

_____

_____

Accomplishments:

_____

_____

_____

_____

_____

chapter

13

Braiding and Braid Extensions

After studying this chapter and completing the Essential Companion *components, you should be able to:*

1. Perform a client consultation with respect to hair braiding.

2. Explain how to prepare the hair for braiding.

3. Demonstrate the procedures for the invisible braid, rope braid, and fishtail braid.

4. Demonstrate the procedures for single braids, with and without extensions.

5. Demonstrate the procedures for cornrowing, with and without extensions.

essential braiding

Why do I need to learn about braiding when I am not interested in providing these services?

Long hairstyles with braids are becoming more and more popular across cultures, generations, and ethnic backgrounds. The fact is that many licensed cosmetologists do not offer these types of services. This can present a problem for clients desiring them. However, it can present an opportunity for those professionals who are expert in these services and readily available to provide them. By offering total hair care services to all clients, you will build a solid client base more readily and will never need to refer a client to another stylist or salon. In the end, you will reap the benefits of increased income and satisfied clients.

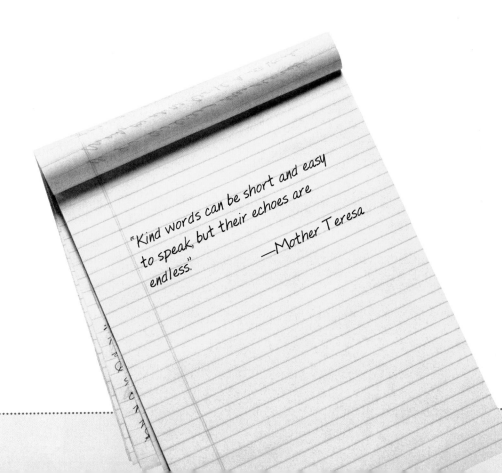

"Kind words can be short and easy to speak, but their echoes are endless."

—Mother Teresa

essential concepts of braiding

What do I need to know about braiding in order to provide a quality service?

In order to be properly prepared to offer quality braiding services, the first step you have to perfect is the client consultation. As with any service, learning to communicate with the client and truly listen to his or her desires, interests, and requests will be key in the success of the service. You will need to learn the important steps in preparing textured hair for a braiding and/or hair extension service. Finally, you will need to be able to demonstrate masterful techniques for a wide variety of braids including invisible, rope, fishtail, and single braids. You will want to perfect your skills in single braids and cornrowing, both with and without extensions. Once you have mastered these skills, you will have taken the first step in establishing a sound braiding business.

essential experience

1

Preparing Textured Hair for Braiding

Number the following steps in their proper procedural order.

_____ Wash your hands.

_____ Gently towel-dry the hair.

_____ Gather required implements, materials, and supplies.

_____ Part damp hair from ear to ear across the crown. Use butterfly clips to separate the front section for back section.

_____ Shampoo, rinse, apply conditioner, and rinse thoroughly.

_____ Part back of head into four to six sections. Separate the sections with clips.

_____ Perform a client consultation and hair/scalp analysis.

_____ Beginning on the left section in the back, start combing the ends of the hair first, working your way up to the base of scalp. Lightly spray the section as you go along with detangling solution, if needed.

_____ Open one of the combed sections. Using fingers, apply blow-drying cream to hair from scalp to ends.

_____ Repeat steps 4 and 5 with the other sections of the hair until the entire head is sectioned.

_____ After combing thoroughly, divide section into two equal parts and twist them together to the end and hold section in place.

_____ Blow-dry using a pick nozzle attachment and hold hair down and away from the client's head as you begin drying. Use comb-out motion with the pick, always pointing the nozzle away from client.

_____ Place client under a medium heat hood dryer for five to ten minutes to remove excess moisture.

_____ Drape the client for a shampoo. If necessary, comb and detangle the hair.

essential
2 experience

The Developmental Stages of Locks

In the space provided, list all five phases in the development of locks in the left column. In the right column, thoroughly explain each phase.

STAGE	DEVELOPMENT

essential
experience
3

Procedure for Basic Cornrows

Number the following steps in their proper procedural order.

_____ Repeat until all the hair is braided. Apply oil sheen for a finished look.

_____ Gather and arrange required materials, implements, and supplies.

_____ To create a panel, start by taking two even partings to form a neat row for the cornrow base. With a tail comb, part the hair into a panel, using butterfly clips to keep the other hair pinned to either side.

_____ As you move along the braid panel, pick up a strand from the scalp with each revolution and add it to the outer strand before crossing it under, alternating the side of the braid on which you pick up the hair.

_____ Divide the panel into three even strands. To ensure consistency, make sure strands are the same size. Place fingers close to the base. Cross the left strand (1) under the center strand (2). The center strand is now on the left and strand 1 is the new center.

_____ Shampoo and condition the client's hair, then comb and blow-dry. If the client has shampooed hair at home, brush hair with a paddle brush.

_____ Cross the right strand (3) under the center strand (1). Passing the outer strands under the center strand this way creates the underhand cornrow braid.

_____ Place capes and towels in the hamper for laundering.

_____ With each crossing under, or revolution, pick up from the base of the panel a new strand of equal size and add it to the outer strand before crossing it under the center strand.

_____ Depending on desired style, determine the correct size and direction of the cornrow base. With tail comb, part hair into two-inch sections and apply a light essential oil to the scalp. Massage oil throughout scalp and hair.

_____ As new strands are added, the braid will become fuller. Braid to the end.

(continued)

essential
3 experience *continued*

_____ Simply braiding to the ends can finish the cornrow; small rubber bands can be used to hold the ends in place.

_____ Braid the next panel in the same direction and in the same manner. Keep the partings clean and even.

_____ Wash your hands with soap and warm water.

_____ Disinfect all implements.

_____ Sanitize your workstation.

essential
4 experience

Word Search

After determining the correct words from the clues provided, locate the words in the word search puzzle.

_____ Occurs after several years of maturation of a lock

_____ Another name for cornrows

_____ Narrow rows of visible braids that lie close to the scalp

_____ Flat leather pads with close and fine teeth

_____ Another name for locks

_____ Simple, two-strand braid in which hair is picked up from the sides and added to the strands as they are crossed over each other

_____ The stage when a bulb can be felt at the end of each lock

_____ A board of fine, upright nails

_____ Another name for visible braid

_____ Three-strand braid produced by overlapping the strands of hair on top of each other

_____ A manufactured synthetic fiber similar to coiled hair types

_____ Beautiful wool fiber from Africa

_____ Natural textured hair that is intertwined and meshed together to form a single or separate network

_____ The phase of lock development when the lock is totally closed on the end

_____ This method of locking takes advantage of the hair's natural ability to coil

_____ In this stage of development, the hair is soft and coiled into spiral configurations

_____ Braid made with two strands that are twisted around each other

_____ Free-hanging braids, with or without extensions, that can be executed either underhand or overhand

_____ This is the lock development stage where hair beings to interlace and mesh

_____ This refers to the hair diameter, feel, and wave pattern

_____ Three-strand braid made by the underhand technique

_____ Strong fiber from ox

```
I  L  R  D  D  A  G  N  I  W  O  R  G  X  Y
N  S  P  R  O  U  T  I  N  G  L  S  F  S  H
V  U  R  A  B  A  S  L  V  A  W  I  I  F  P
I  U  E  O  D  V  E  O  E  O  S  N  N  T  O
S  L  -  B  D  R  H  E  R  H  G  Q  O  J  R
I  M  L  G  X  Y  E  N  T  L  R  C  L  C  T
B  A  O  N  X  D  R  A  E  B  P  Z  A  A  A
L  T  C  I  W  O  I  B  D  U  P  U  K  N  L
E  U  K  W  C  L  R  A  B  L  H  M  E  E  W
B  R  S  A  B  A  E  F  R  H  O  Y  N  R  W
R  A  I  R  I  N  N  H  A  B  A  C  A  O  M
A  T  A  D  O  G  P  Z  I  K  E  C  K  W  H
I  I  S  P  T  I  S  M  D  J  X  P  K  S  E
D  O  I  M  Y  I  B  P  A  L  M  R  O  L  L
N  N  S  I  O  P  Y  G  T  E  X  T  U  R  E
```

essential
experience
5

Research and Design

- Contact various salons in your area and interview them by asking the following questions.
  a) Does your salon offer braiding and/or extensions as a service?
  b) If yes, what braiding services do you offer?
  c) What braids are the most popular in your salon?
  d) What is the average time it takes your stylists to complete a full head of cornrows?
  e) What is the price structure your salon charges for braiding services?
  f) Do you have any specific advice for a newly licensed professional with respect to offering braiding services?

- Look through various style magazines and locate at least three different braided styles. Recreate those styles on a mannequin or a model.

- Use your imagination and the skills you have mastered in braiding to create a special effects braid. Stylists have created such looks as hats, flowers, baskets, or bird cages with braids. Tap into your creative abilities and design your own special look.

essential review

Using the following words, fill in the blanks below to form a thorough review of Chapter 13, "Braiding and Braid Extensions." Words or terms may be used more than once or not at all.

box braids	diffuser	network	round
center strand	double twisting	occupation	several weeks
challenges	forehead	oval	shorter
chemicals	jawline	ox	small forehead
coil	length	palm roll	softens
coil pattern	locks	partial bangs	spiral
cornrows	matte finish	pomades	configurations
dampened	maturation	rope	synthetic fiber
subsections	nails	ropelike	temples
diameter	natural curl	rotating motion	visible

1. Braiding styles have been known to distinguish one's tribe, age, economic status, _____, geographic location, religious standing, and marital status.

2. Hair is referred to as "natural" or "virgin" if it has had no previous coloring or lightening treatments, _____, or physical abuse.

3. Natural hairstyling uses no chemicals or tints and does not alter the _____ or coil pattern of the hair.

4. When referring to braiding and other natural hairstyling, the term *texture* refers to the _____ of the hair, the wave pattern of the hair, and the feel of the hair.

5. With regard to wave pattern, a _____ is a very tight curl pattern that is spiral in formation and, when lengthened or stretched, resembles a series of loops.

6. When styling with braids, add height to create the illusion of thinness for the _____facial shape.

7. Most braided styles are appropriate for the _____ facial shape.

8. Create styles that are full around the forehead or _____ to help create a more oval appearance for the diamond facial shape.

9. To create the illusion of length and to soften facial lines for the square facial shape, choose styles that frame the face around the _____, temples, and jawline.

essential review *continued*

10. Soft fringes around the forehead will camouflage a _____ without closing up the triangular-shaped face.

11. Creating full styles can make the oblong face shape appear _____ or wider.

12. The goals for the inverted triangle face shape is to minimize the width of the forehead by styling with _____ or wisps of hair/braids that frame the face.

13. A natural hairbrush, also known as a boar-bristle brush, is best for stimulating the scalp as well as removing dirt and lint from _____ .

14. The tool that dries the hair without disturbing the finished look and without removing moisture is called a _____ .

15. A board made of fine, upright _____ through which human hair extensions are combed is called a hackle.

16. A manufactured _____ of excellent quality that has a texture similar to curly or coiled hair is called kanekalon.

17. A beautiful wool fiber imported from Africa which has a _____ and comes only in black and brown is known as lin.

18. A strong fiber that comes from the domestic _____ found in the mountains of Tibet and Central Asia is yak.

19. _____ , gels, or lotions can be used to hold the hair in place for a finished look.

20. Textured hair, or hair with a tight _____ , presents certain challenges when styling because it is very fragile when both wet and dry.

21. Blow-drying the hair _____ it, makes it more manageable, loosens it, and elongates the wave pattern while stretching the hair shaft length.

22. Another term for a _____ braid is inverted.

23. The inverted braid is a three-strand braid that employs the underhand technique, in which strands of hair are woven under the _____ .

24. A _____ braid is made with two strands that are twisted around each other.

25. Single braids, _____ , and individual braids are all considered to be free-hanging braids, with or without extensions, that can be extended with either an underhand or overhand stitch.

26. Narrow, visible braids that lie close to the scalp are called _____ .

27. There are several ways to cultivate locks such as _____ , wrapping with cord, coiling, braiding, or simply by not combing or brushing.

essential review *continued*

28. Dreadlocks are natural textured hair that is intertwined and meshed together to form a single or separate _____ of hair and is done without the use of chemicals.

29. The method of placing the comb at the base of the scalp and, with a _____, spiraling the hair into a curl is known as the comb technique.

30. The method that involves applying gel to _____, placing the portion of hair between the palms of both hands, and rolling in a circular direction is known as palm roll.

31. Braids or extensions are an effective way to start locks. They involve sectioning the hair for the desired lock and single braiding the hair to the end, with or without adding hair extensions, and waiting for _____ of growth before employing the palm roll technique.

32. During the maturation stage of locks, the lock is totally closed at the end and the hair is tightly meshed, giving a _____ cylinder shape, except where there is new growth at the base.

33. During the pre-lock stage of locks, the hair is soft and coiled into _____ that are smooth and with open ends.

essential discoveries and accomplishments

In the space below, jot some notes about what concepts of this chapter were hardest for you to understand or remember. Imagine finding yourself suddenly in the role of "teacher" and consider what you would tell your "students" about these difficult concepts.

Share your *Essential Discoveries* with some of the other students in your class and ask if they are helpful to them. You may want to revise your notes based on good ideas shared by your peers. Under "Accomplishments," list at least three things you have accomplished since your last entry that relate to your career goals.

Discoveries:

_____

_____

_____

_____

_____

Accomplishments:

_____

_____

_____

_____

_____

_____

Wigs and Hair Enhancements

essential objectives

After studying this chapter and completing the Essential Companion *components, you should be able to:*

1. List the elements of a client consultation for wig services.

2. Explain the differences between human-hair and synthetic wigs.

3. Describe the two basic categories of wigs.

4. Demonstrate the procedure for taking wig measurements.

5. Demonstrate the procedure for putting on a wig.

6. Describe the various types of hairpieces and their uses.

7. Explain the various methods of attaching extensions.

essential
aspects of wigs and hair enhancements

Do people really still wear wigs? Why should I know how to handle them?

Yes, people really do still wear wigs. They wear them for a number of reasons—from convenience to hair loss. Celebrities and people in the public eye, both male and female, wear wigs, hairpieces, or toupees regularly to create a different, dramatic look. Like many other cosmetology services you will learn, the use of wigs has been prevalent throughout history from the early Egyptians to the present time. They became extremely popular again in the mid-twentieth century and continue to be used extensively in theater, music and movie productions today.

From time to time, you will also have clients who have medical problems or are undergoing chemotherapy treatments. As a result they may experience partial or total hair loss and will want to use wigs to maintain their personal appearance. You will need to be prepared to provide them the quality service they deserve, especially if they are experiencing a difficult time.

essential concepts in the artistry of artificial hair

What can really be so hard about handling wigs, and what do I really need to know?

You need to know about the construction and materials used in wigs and how to care for each type of product, whether it is a human hair piece or one constructed of synthetic hair. It will be important for you to know how to properly measure a client's head size and fit a wig. You will also want to master the special care needed for human-hair and hand-knotted wigs. Hairpieces are an increasingly popular salon service, and by learning different attachment methods you can offer clients an even wider variety of services.

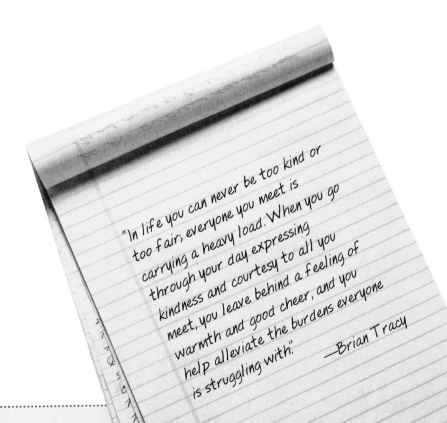

"In life you can never be too kind or too fair; everyone you meet is carrying a heavy load. When you go through your day expressing kindness and courtesy to all you meet, you leave behind a feeling of warmth and good cheer, and you help alleviate the burdens everyone is struggling with."

—Brian Tracy

essential experience

1

The History of Wigs

Research the history of wigs and write a brief essay on the subject. Be prepared to present the report to the full class if directed by your instructor. There are a number of resources you can refer, including your school's library or resource center, encyclopedias, the Internet, and the community library. Obtain copies of pictures and prepare drawings to help illustrate your report.

_____

_____

_____

_____

_____

_____

_____

_____

_____

_____

_____

_____

_____

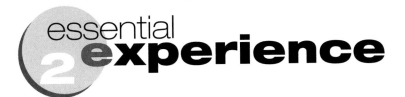

essential 2 experience

Wig Measurements

Locate at least five models and measure their heads for a wig. Use the following chart to record your findings.

Model Name					
Circumference					
Middle of Forehead to Nape					
Ear to Ear across Forehead					
Ear to Ear over Top of Head					
Temple to Temple across Crown					
Width at Nape Line across Nape of Neck					

essential
experience
3

Matching Exercise

Match each of the following essential terms with its definition.

_____ Turned hair

_____ Fusion

_____ Weft

_____ Capless wig

_____ Block

_____ Hairpiece

_____ Hand-tied wig

_____ Hair extensions

_____ Cap wig

_____ Bonding

1. Method of attaching hair extensions in which hair wefts or single strands are attached with adhesive or a glue gun.

2. Strip of human or artificial hair woven by hand or machine onto a thread.

3. Wig made by inserting individual strands of hair into a mesh foundation and knotting them with a needle.

4. Hair in which the roots and hair ends of all strands are aligned so that the cuticles slope in the same direction.

5. Wig consisting of elasticized mesh-fiber base to which the hair is attached.

6. Hair additions that are secured to the base of the client's natural hair in order to add length, volume, texture, or color.

7. Small wig that covers the top or crown of the head.

8. Head-shaped form, usually made of canvas-covered cork or Styrofoam, to which the wig is secured for fitting, cleaning, coloring, and styling.

9. A machine-made wig in which rows of wefts are sewn to elastic strips in a circular pattern to fit the head shape.

10. Method of attaching extensions in which the extension hair is bonded to the client's own hair with a bonding material that is activated by heat from a special tool.

essential experience
4

Crossword Puzzle

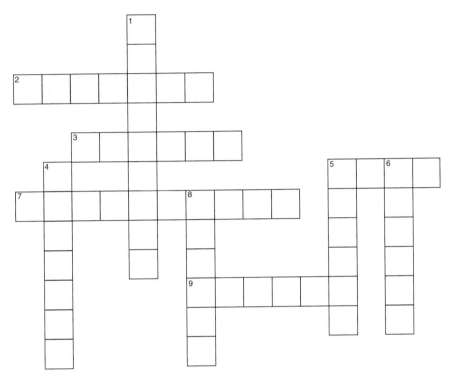

Across

2. Method of attaching hair extensions with adhesive or glue gun
3. Wig consisting of elasticized mesh fiber to which hair is attached
5. Strip of hair woven by hand or machine onto a thread
7. Machine-made wig
9. Small wig used to cover top or crown of a man's head

Down

1. Hair addition that sits on top of hair and is usually attached by temporary methods
4. Hairpiece with an oblong base and curls or cluster of curls
5. Hairpiece that fits on the top or back of head
6. Method of attaching extensions with bonding material activated by heat
8. Hairpiece consisting of a long length of wefted hair mounted with a loop on the end

essential
5 experience

Windowpaning—Wig Care

Windowpaning is the process of transferring key elements, points, or steps in a lesson into visual images that are hand sketched into the squares or "panes" of a matrix. Let your mind think in pictures and sketch the essential concepts printed in each of the following windowpanes. Don't be concerned with your artistic ability. Use lines and stick figures to depict the concepts requested.

Measure Circumference of Head	**Measure Over Top to Nape**	**Measure from Ear to Ear across Forehead**
Measure from Ear to Over Top of Head	**Measure from Temple to Temple across Crown**	**Measure Width of Napeline**
Test for Human Hair	**Placement of T-pins**	**Cascade**

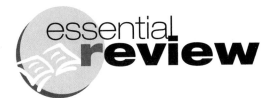

essential **review**

Using the following words, fill in the blanks below to form a thorough review of Chapter 14, "Wigs and Hair Enhancements." Words or terms may be used more than once or not at all.

40 percent	bronze razors	fusion	six
60 percent	cap wigs	hand-tied	split
70 percent	capless wigs	human-hair	strand test
adhesive	cuticle-intact	integration	synthetic
angora	eight	key point checklist	ten
attitudinal	emotional	machine-made	toupee
boar bristles	film	oxidizing	track and sew
bonding	free-form	pin curls	wig

1. The ancient Egyptians shaved their heads with _____ and wore heavy wigs to protect them from the sun.

2. A wig service can be a large financial and _____ investment for a client.

3. Your best tool for achieving good communication during a wig consultation is to follow the _____.

4. A _____ can be defined as an artificial covering for the head consisting of a network of interwoven hair.

5. One advantage of _____ wigs is that they have the same styling and maintenance requirements as natural hair.

6. One disadvantage of human hair wigs is that the hair will break and _____ just like human hair if mistreated by harsh brushing, back-combing, or excessive use of heat.

7. Most _____, ready-to-wear wigs are cut according to the latest styles, with the cut, color, and texture already set.

8. Well-crafted wigs, such as those used in _____ work, might be valued at thousands of dollars.

9. Animal hair that may be mixed with human hair to create a wig includes _____, horse, yak, or sheep hair.

essential review *continued*

10. Hair that has been "turned" is also known as _____ hair.

11. _____ are constructed with an elasticized mesh-fiber base to which the hair is attached.

12. _____ are machine-made with the hair woven into long strips called wefts.

13. _____ wigs are made by inserting individual strands of hair into a mesh foundation and knotting them with a needle.

14. Two ways to prepare the hair for a wig are with _____ and by wrapping the hair.

15. Canvas wig blocks are available in _____ sizes.

16. _____ cutting is usually done on dry hair, which allows you to see more clearly how the hair will fall.

17. Traditionally, brushes made with natural _____ have been regarded as the best on human hair.

18. Do not use _____ haircolor or haircolor with peroxide on wig hair that has been treated with metallic hair dye.

19. When coloring wigs or hairpieces, always _____ the hair prior to full color application.

20. A hairpiece gives 20 percent to _____ coverage and sits on top of the hair.

21. _____ hairpieces are very lightweight, natural-looking, add length and volume to the client's hair, and allow the client's own hair to be pulled through and blended with the hair of the hairpiece.

22. A _____ is a small wig used to cover the top and crown of the head.

23. A method of attaching hair extensions that requires certification training is _____ .

24. In the bonding method, hair extensions are attached with _____ .

25. In the _____ method, hair extensions are secured at the base of the client's own hair by sewing.

essential discoveries and accomplishments

In the space below, jot some notes about what concepts of this chapter were hardest for you to understand or remember. Imagine finding yourself suddenly in the role of "teacher" and consider what you would tell your "students" about these difficult concepts.

Share your *Essential Discoveries* with some of the other students in your class and ask if they are helpful to them. You may want to revise your notes based on good ideas shared by your peers. Under "Accomplishments," list at least three things you have accomplished since your last entry that relate to your career goals.

Discoveries:

_____

_____

_____

_____

_____

_____

Accomplishments:

_____

_____

_____

_____

_____

_____

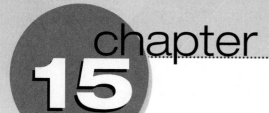

chapter

15

Chemical Texture Services

essential
objectives

After studying this chapter and completing the Essential
Companion *components, you should be able to:*

1. List the elements of a hair analysis for chemical texture services.

2. Explain the physical and chemical actions that take place during permanent waving.

3. List and describe the various types of permanent waving solutions.

4. Demonstrate base wrapping procedures: straight set, curvature wrap, bricklay wrap, weave wrap, double tool wrap, and spiral wrap.

5. Describe the procedure for chemical hair relaxing.

6. Explain the basic procedure for soft curl permanent.

essential chemical texture services

What role will permanent waving and hair relaxing play in my career when all I really want to do is style hair?

Actually, permanent waving, also known as a texture service, is the most popular chemical service offered in salons today. You will find that being able to provide your client with an appropriate texture service will improve your effectiveness as a hair designer. People have been trying to change the wave patterns of their hair since ancient Roman and Egyptian civilizations. Women wrapped their hair around sticks, and men wove their beards around them and then applied river mud, which they allowed to dry in the sun for up to three days to achieve the desired look.

We've come a long way since those primitive methods. We began to make real progress in the first part of the twentieth century when Charles Nessler invented the permanent wave machine. Then, in 1931, the pre-heat method of perming was introduced, followed the next year by a method using external heat generated by chemical reaction. By 1941, the cold wave method was invented, which used chemicals to soften and expand the hair and then re-harden it in its newly formed shape. This method does not use heat in any form. Technology continues to improve and new products are introduced regularly which allow the professional cosmetologist to modify the wave pattern of a client's hair and render it more suitable for the desired style.

Our client culture has changed dramatically in the last few decades. Clients today want instant gratification from their salon visit, and nearly all want more manageable hair. A texture service can play a huge role in helping the client manage his/her personal style between visits to the salon. Relaxers remove wave or curl from the hair in varying degrees. There is a large variety of hair types, as well as individuals who want the curl in their hair reduced. Hair relaxing services generate significant revenue for you and the salon. As a professional, you will want to be fully prepared to offer a quality service when it is requested.

essential concepts of chemical texture services

Exactly what am I going to need to learn about permanent waving and chemical hair relaxing to be considered competent in these particular skills?

Your success in chemical texture services depends on your knowledge of the hair, your understanding of the chemicals used, and your ability to physically perform the service. Other factors relevant to the success of the service include the condition or integrity of the hair. The professional cosmetologist will know how to properly analyze a client's hair and scalp and select the appropriate products to create the desired look. You will also need to know how to select the correct tools and how to properly use them to "set" the perm. In addition, you need to prescribe the proper care of the chemical service to maintain its look for the maximum period of time.

Research and development of relaxer systems continues daily. As a result, we see state-of-the-art formulas and products available for our use in the salon. You will be exposed to these formulas while you are in school as well as in the professional establishment. Many of the manufacturers provide excellent education in the use of their products, and you will want to take advantage of all the information that is available to you. In addition to product technology, you will want to learn about the tools used in relaxing treatments as well as the procedures to follow to ensure success. As in perming, you must learn to conduct a thorough client consultation complete with hair and scalp analysis. Finally, you must master all the safety precautions which must be followed in this critical service.

"It is not because things are difficult that we do not dare, it is because we do not dare that they are difficult."
—Seneca

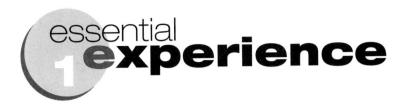

essential experience 1

Defining Permanent Waving and Identifying Wave Patterns

Permanent waving is a chemical and physical process in which the hair is wrapped around a rod, chemically softened and expanded, and finally chemically rehardened into its newly formed shape.

In order to better understand the concept of wave patterns, look through old magazines (not beauty-industry related) for examples of different types. You are not looking for patterns that involve human hair. Cut out examples of wave and curl patterns (such as ocean waves) and paste them below, creating a collage. Beneath the collage, write a brief narrative describing the various patterns selected and how they differ from each other.

_____

_____

_____

_____

essential
2 experience

Hair Analysis

Perform a complete consultation and hair analysis on three other students in your class. Complete the school's client record card for each student. Determine the correct rod size and product choice to create their desired textured look. Ask your instructor to review your record card and make an assessment about the results you might achieve.

essential
3 experience

Product Research

Research the various perm products used in your school. Make a chart of the products listing name, pH, key ingredients, and hair type for which they are recommended.

Product Name	Product pH	Key Ingredients	Hair Type

essential
4 experience

Matching

Match the following essential terms with their identifying phrase or definition.

_____	Coarse texture	**1.** Result of overprocessing
_____	Cortex	**2.** Smaller partings, small-to-medium size rods
_____	Cuticle	**3.** Smaller partings, larger rods
_____	Fine texture	**4.** Normal hair
_____	Good porosity	**5.** Resistant hair
_____	Medium texture	**6.** Innermost section of the hair
_____	Medulla	**7.** Average size partings, medium rods
_____	Overporous	**8.** Outer covering of the hair
_____	Poor porosity	**9.** Major component of the hair structure
_____	Underprocessing	**10.** Gives support to style without definite curl
_____	Plastic cap	**11.** One end paper folded over hair strand
_____	Elasticity	**12.** Shorter hair wound from ends toward scalp
_____	Density	**13.** The number of hairs per square inch
_____	Body wave	**14.** The ability of the hair to stretch and contract
_____	Waving lotion	**15.** Porous papers used to cover hair ends
_____	Bookend wrap	**16.** Heat is created chemically within the product
_____	Exothermic	**17.** Fits over the wrapped rods
_____	Croquignole	**18.** Amino acids are bonded together and form these
_____	End wraps	**19.** Caused by insufficient processing time
_____	Polypeptides	**20.** A liquid that softens and expands the hair shaft

essential
5 experience

Product Research

Research a variety of relaxer products available in your school and found at local supply stores. Use the chart below to track your findings.

Product Name	Sodium or Thio?	Is a Base Required?	What Is the Percentage of Sodium Hydroxide?	What Is the pH?	For What Hair Type Is the Product Used?

essential experience

6

Purpose and Action of Chemical Hair Relaxing

List the products used in chemical hair relaxers.

_____

_____

In your own words, explain the action of sodium hydroxide on the hair.

_____

_____

_____

_____

_____

What is the common ingredient in a thio type relaxer and permanent waving solution?

_____

Explain the action of this common ingredient.

_____

_____

What is the purpose of the neutralizer in chemical relaxing treatments?

_____

_____

_____

In your own words, explain the difference between base and "no-base" formulas, and the purpose of using a base product.

_____

_____

_____

_____

_____

_____

essential
experience
7

Word Search

After determining the correct words from the clues provided, locate the words in the word search puzzle.

Word	Clue
_____	Perm type having a pH between 7.8 and 8.2
_____	Perm type having a pH between 9.0 and 9.6
_____	Oily cream used to protect the skin and scalp during hair relaxing
_____	Perm wrap in which one end paper is folded in half over hair ends
_____	Rod having a smaller circumference in the center than on the ends
_____	Hair strands are wrapped from ends to scalp
_____	Partings and bases radiate throughout the panels to follow the curvature of the head
_____	Side bonds between the polypeptide chains in the cortex
_____	Waves activated by an outside heat source
_____	Relatively weak physical side bonds resulting from an attraction between opposite electrical charges
_____	Process by which hydroxide relaxers permanently straighten hair
_____	Process of stopping the action of the permanent wave solution and hardening hair in new form
_____	Also called end bonds
_____	Relaxer having a pH above 10 and a higher concentration of ammonium thioglycolate
_____	Wrapping technique that uses zigzag partings to divide base areas

```
G  N  C  E  Q  C  U  N  O  H  E  Y  E  D  S
H  E  O  N  W  U  B  O  J  F  R  I  S  M  D
Y  N  N  I  I  R  X  I  R  J  F  S  B  C  N
D  D  C  L  T  V  S  T  B  V  U  O  A  R  O
R  O  A  A  F  A  U  A  S  L  O  M  S  O  B
O  T  V  K  B  T  Z  Z  F  K  P  H  E  Q  E
G  H  E  L  K  U  P  I  E  B  O  W  C  U  D
E  E  R  A  M  R  D  N  L  V  C  A  R  I  I
N  R  O  S  X  E  D  O  T  A  O  O  E  G  T
B  M  D  G  B  W  Y  I  W  M  R  L  A  N  P
O  I  T  O  R  R  Z  H  U  E  J  T  M  O  E
N  C  N  A  F  A  D  T  Z  P  A  Q  U  L  P
D  D  P  O  E  P  G  N  B  D  K  V  B  E  I
S  A  C  I  D  -  B  A  L  A  N  C  E  D  N
F  N  N  R  E  X  A  L  E  R  O  I  H  T  X
```

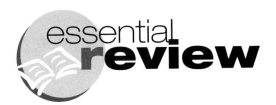

Complete the following review of Chapter 15, "Chemical Texture Services," by circling the correct answer to each question.

1. _____ rods have a small diameter in the center area and gradually increase to their largest diameter at the ends, resulting in a tighter curl at hair ends, with a loose, wider curl at the scalp.

   a) convex　　　　　　　　　　b) straight

   c) concave　　　　　　　　　　d) colored

2. A method of wrapping a permanent wave that is suitable for very long hair is the

   _____ .

   a) double halo method　　　　b) double tool technique

   c) single halo method　　　　d) straight back method

3. A _____ is an example of a physical change that results from breaking and re-forming the hydrogen bonds within the hair.

   a) blow-dry service　　　　　b) wet set

   c) hair color service　　　　　d) comb-out

4. All perm wraps begin by sectioning the hair into panels which are further divided into subsections called _____ .

   a) panels　　　　　　　　　　b) base sections

   c) base panels　　　　　　　　d) base control

5. Always rinse perm solution from the hair for at least _____ minutes before applying the neutralizer.

   a) two　　　　　　　　　　　b) three

   c) four　　　　　　　　　　　d) five

6. A/an _____ liquid protein conditioner can be applied to the hair and dried under a warm dryer for five minutes or more prior to neutralization if hair is damaged.

   a) alkaline　　　　　　　　　b) emulsified

   c) neutral　　　　　　　　　　d) acidic

7. Ask _____ to find out why the client wants the texture service and what results are expected.

   a) open-ended questions　　　b) closed-ended questions

   c) rhetorical questions　　　　d) personal questions

essential review *continued*

8. Base control refers to the position of the tool in relation to its _____ and is determined by the angle at which the hair is wrapped.

a) panel

b) base section

c) base panel

d) scalp position

9. End wraps are absorbent papers used to _____ of the hair when wrapping and winding hair on the perm tools.

a) decrease the moisture

b) control the ends

c) control the elasticity

d) decrease the elasticity

10. Hair texture describes the _____ of a single strand of hair and is classified as fine, medium, or coarse.

a) length

b) color

c) curl

d) diameter

11. If the hair is not _____, the hydrogen peroxide in the neutralizer can react with waving lotion and cause the hair color to lighten.

a) thoroughly shampooed

b) rinsed properly

c) lightly shampooed

d) lightly rinsed

12. If too many _____ bonds are broken in the perming process, the hair will be too weak to hold a firm curl.

a) disulfide

b) hydrogen

c) salt

d) polypeptide

13. If you suspect metallic salts are present, mix one ounce of 20 volume peroxide with twenty drops of 28 percent _____ and immerse at least twenty strands for thirty minutes.

a) bleach

b) hydrogen

c) ammonia

d) petroleum

14. If hair breaks under very slight strain, it has:

a) excellent elasticity

b) very good elasticity

c) average elasticity

d) little or no elasticity

15. In order to make a smooth transition from the rolled section of the head to an unrolled section, use a larger tool for the last tool next to an unrolled section when giving a

_____ .

a) curvature perm

b) partial perm

c) spiral perm

d) full perm

essential review *continued*

16. In neutralization, the bonds in the hair are re-formed _____ .

a) immediately

b) slowly

c) sporadically

d) randomly

17. In permanent waving, most of the processing takes place as soon as the solution penetrates the hair, within the first _____ minutes.

a) one to two

b) two to three

c) three to four

d) five to ten

18. Many male clients are looking for added _____, style, and low maintenance that only a perm can provide.

a) color

b) shine

c) fullness

d) length

19. Metallic salts leave a coating on the hair that may cause _____, severe discoloration, or hair breakage.

a) mild odor

b) uneven curls

c) calcification

d) smooth curls

20. Neutralization rebuilds the _____ by removing the extra hydrogen bonds created by the waving solution.

a) salt bonds

b) hydrogen bonds

c) disulfide bonds

d) polypeptide chains

21. Perming only a section of a whole head of hair is called _____ .

a) section perming

b) spotmatic perming

c) partial perming

d) limited perming

22. Some manufacturers recommend the application of a _____ after blotting and before application of the neutralizer.

a) pre-neutralizing conditioner

b) pre-neutralizing shampoo

c) post-processing moisturizer

d) post-processing shampoo

23. The _____ wrap uses zigzag partings to divide base areas.

a) curvature perm

b) weave technique

c) bricklay perm

d) straight perm

24. The _____ wrap creates a movement that curves within sectioned-out panels.

a) curvature perm

b) bricklay perm

c) weave technique

d) straight perm

essential review *continued*

25. The basic perm wrap is also called a _____ wrap.

    a) curvature perm   b) bricklay perm

    c) weave technique   d) straight set

26. The chemical action of _____ breaks the disulfide bonds and softens the hair.

    a) ammonia   b) hydrogen peroxide

    c) waving lotion   d) neutralizer

27. The chemical composition of hair consists almost entirely of a protein material called

_____ .

    a) polypeptides   b) keratin

    c) cysteine   d) melanin

28. Bonds that are formed between two cysteine amino acids, located on neighboring polypeptide chains, are:

    a) salt   b) chemical

    c) hydrogen   d) disulfide

29. The polypeptide chains of this layer of hair are connected by end bonds and cross-linked by side bonds that form the fibers and structure of hair.

    a) medulla   b) cuticle

    c) cortex   d) follicle

30. The perm that is activated by heat created chemically within the product is known

as _____ .

    a) endothermic   b) alkaline

    c) exothermic   d) sodium hydroxide

31. The action of waving lotion is to _____ .

    a) discolor the hair   b) shrink the hair

    c) expand the hair   d) condition the hair

32. The degree to which hair absorbs the waving lotion is related to its _____ .

    a) texture   b) length

    c) elasticity   d) porosity

33. The length of time required for the hair strands to absorb the waving lotion and for the hair to re-curl is called _____ .

    a) application time   b) processing time

    c) rinsing time   d) development time

essential review *continued*

34. The main active ingredient in acid-balanced waving lotions is _____ .

   a) glyceryl monothioglycolate   b) ammonium thioglycolate

   c) hydrogen peroxide   d) sodium hydroxide

35. The main active ingredient or reducing agent in alkaline perms is _____ .

   a) glycerol monothioglycolate   b) ammonium thioglycolate

   c) hydrogen peroxide   d) sodium hydroxide

36. The _____ wrap is used to prevent noticeable splits and to blend the flow of the hair.

   a) curvature perm   b) bricklay perm

   c) spiral perm   d) basic perm

37. The _____ wrap is done at an angle that causes the hair to spiral along the length of the tool, like the grip on a tennis racquet.

   a) spiral   b) croquignole

   c) bricklay   d) barber pole

38. The hydrogen atoms in the disulfide bonds are so strongly attracted to the oxygen in the neutralizer that they release their bond with the sulfur atoms and join with the

_____ .

   a) salt bond   b) nitrogen

   c) hydrogen   d) oxygen

39. Underprocessing is caused by _____ processing time of the waving lotion.

   a) excessive   b) increasing

   c) insufficient   d) exact

40. Waves that process more quickly and produce firmer curls than true acid waves are considered to be _____ .

   a) alkaline   b) acid-balanced

   c) ammonium thioglycolate   d) sodium hydroxide

41. What can be used to determine the actual processing time needed to achieve optimum curl results when giving a perm for the first time on a client?

   a) patch test   b) strand test

   c) porosity test   d) preliminary test curl

42. What type of hair is more fragile, easier to process, and more susceptible to damage from perm services?

   a) coarse texture   b) medium texture

   c) non-elastic   d) fine texture

essential review *continued*

43. What type of hair requires more processing than medium or fine hair and may also be more resistant to processing?

a) coarse texture

b) medium texture

c) non-elastic

d) fine texture

44. When the strand of hair is wrapped at an angle 45 degrees beyond perpendicular to its base section, it will result in _____ .

a) half-off base placement

b) off-base placement

c) on-base placement

d) on-stem placement

45. When one end paper is folded in half over the hair ends like an envelope, it is called the _____ .

a) double end paper wrap

b) book end wrap

c) single end paper wrap

d) top-hand wrap

46. When the strand of hair is wrapped at an angle 90 degrees (perpendicular) to its base section, it will result in:

a) half-off base placement

b) off-base placement

c) on-base placement

d) on-stem placement

47. When performing a procedure for a preliminary test curl, wrap one tool in each different area of the head including the top, the side, and the _____ .

a) bang

b) temple

c) nape

d) occipital

48. When hair has assumed the desired shape, the broken disulfide bonds must be _____ rebonded.

a) chemically

b) physically

c) temporarily

d) semi-permanently

49. When you place one end wrap on top of the hair strand and hold it flat, it is called the _____ .

a) double flat wrap

b) bookend wrap

c) single flat wrap

d) top-hand wrap

50. A hair relaxing treatment should be avoided when an examination shows the presence of _____ .

a) scalp abrasions

b) strong curl

c) excessive oils

d) pityriasis steadoides

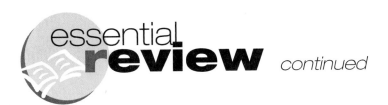
essential **review** *continued*

51. After saturating the rods with neutralizer in a soft curl permanent, the next step is to

_____ .

a) rinse with hot water

b) remove rods carefully

c) completely dry hair

d) apply protective base

52. After the hair has been processed with a sodium hydroxide relaxer and before the shampoo, the hair should be thoroughly:

a) oiled

b) rinsed

c) dried

d) conditioned

53. Before giving a relaxing treatment to overly curly hair, the cosmetologist must judge its texture, porosity and _____ .

a) length and elasticity

b) elasticity and silkiness

c) elasticity and extent of damage, if any

d) softness and extent of damage, if any

54. If using a "no base" relaxer, it is recommended that a protective cream be applied

_____ .

a) at the nape of the neck

b) over the ear lobes

c) at the frontal hairline

d) on the hairline and around the ears

55. Inspecting the action of the relaxer by stretching the strands to see how fast the natural curls are being removed is called _____ .

a) periodic patch testing

b) periodic relaxer testing

c) periodic strand testing

d) periodic elasticity testing

56. Of the general types of hair relaxers, which one does not require pre-shampooing?

a) sodium hydroxide

b) sodium thioglycolate

c) ammonium thioglycolate

d) acid-based relaxers

57. One safety precaution for hair relaxing is to avoid _____ the scalp with the comb or fingernails.

a) massaging

b) scratching

c) smoothing

d) stimulating

58. Relaxers which are ionic compounds formed by a metal which is combined with oxygen and hydrogen are known as _____ .

a) guanidine hydroxide relaxers

b) metal hydroxide relaxers

c) low-pH relaxers

d) no-base relaxers

essential review *continued*

59. Sodium hydroxide relaxers are commonly called _____ .

a) guanidine hydroxide relaxers 　　　b) low pH relaxers

c) lithium hydroxide relaxers 　　　　d) lye relaxers

60. The action of a sodium hydroxide relaxer causes the hair to _____ .

a) soften and swell 　　　　　　　　b) soften and shrink

c) expand and harden 　　　　　　　d) harden and set

61. The process of breaking the hair's disulfide bonds during processing and converting them to lanthionine bonds when the relaxer is rinsed from the hair is known as

_____ .

a) lanolination 　　　　　　　　　　b) lanthionization

c) neutralization 　　　　　　　　　d) normalization

62. The scalp and skin are protected from possible burns when using a hair relaxer by applying _____ .

a) cotton 　　　　　　　　　　　　b) stabilizer

c) base 　　　　　　　　　　　　　d) shampoo

63. The processing time of a chemical relaxer is affected by _____ .

a) styling products used 　　　　　　b) the client's age

c) the hair's porosity 　　　　　　　d) the brand of relaxer

64. The relaxer cream is applied near the scalp last because processing is accelerated in this area by _____ .

a) body heat 　　　　　　　　　　　b) application speed

c) body perspiration 　　　　　　　　d) sebaceous glands

65. The chemical required to stop the action of the chemical relaxer is _____ .

a) petroleum cream 　　　　　　　　b) neutralizer

c) conditioner 　　　　　　　　　　d) waving lotion

66. The best type of shampoo to use after the chemical relaxer is _____ .

a) an organic shampoo 　　　　　　　b) an antibacterial shampoo

c) a neutralizing shampoo 　　　　　　d) a dry shampoo

67. The strength of a relaxer is determined by the strand test. General guidelines suggest that, for coarse virgin hair, the following strength is used.

a) extra mild 　　　　　　　　　　　b) regular

c) mild 　　　　　　　　　　　　　d) strong or super

essential review *continued*

68. The strength of a relaxer is determined by the strand test. General guidelines suggest that for fine, tinted, or lightened hair, the following strength is used.

a) extra mild

b) regular

c) mild

d) strong or super

69. The process of permanently rearranging the basic structure of overly curly hair into a straight form is called _____ .

a) thermal straightening

b) chemical hair relaxing

c) permanent waving

d) chemical hair softening

70. The combination of a thio relaxer and a thio permanent wrapped on large tools is called a _____ .

a) soft curl permanent

b) thioglycolate reconstructer

c) relaxer curl permanent

d) hard curl permanent

71. The most commonly used methods of hair relaxing are the sodium hydroxide method and the _____ method.

a) thermal

b) thio

c) ammonia

d) peroxide

72. To check relaxer processing, smooth and press a strand to the scalp using the back of the comb or your finger. If curl returns, _____ .

a) rinse immediately

b) add neutralizer

c) continue processing

d) add conditioner

73. What is used to restore the hair and scalp to their normal acidic pH?

a) cream conditioner

b) medicated shampoo

c) conditioning filler

d) normalizing lotion

74. What stops the action of any chemical relaxer that may remain in the hair after rinsing?

a) softener

b) breakdown cream

c) swelling compound

d) neutralizer

75. What are the two types of formulas for sodium hydroxide chemical hair relaxers?

a) base and no base

b) lye and no lye

c) stabilizer and no stabilizer

d) cream and no cream

76. What is one safety precaution that must be followed with all chemical hair relaxing services?

a) shampooing the client's hair

b) pre-conditioning the hair

c) advising the client regarding processing time

d) wearing protective gloves

77. What are the three basic steps used in chemical hair relaxing?

a) wrapping, application, rinsing

b) processing, neutralizing, conditioning

c) shampooing, application, conditioning

d) processing, neutralizing, stabilizing

78. When applying sodium hydroxide relaxer, the processing cream is applied last to the
_____ and _____ .

a) scalp area, middle of hair shaft

b) scalp area, hair ends

c) middle of hair shaft, hair ends

d) nape area, hair ends

79. When performing a sodium hydroxide retouch, where is the product applied first?

a) to the hair ends

b) to the new growth only

c) to the middle of the hair shaft

d) to the scalp area only

80. When using the comb method of application, how is the relaxing cream applied?

a) with the back of the comb

b) with the fingers

c) with the applicator brush

d) with the teeth of the comb

81. When processing is complete for a soft curl permanent, what is done after rinsing the hair thoroughly with warm water?

a) each curl is blotted with a towel

b) conditioner is applied

c) client is place under a dryer

d) test curl is taken

82. When hair has been sufficiently straightened, the hair is rinsed rapidly and thoroughly with
_____ water.

a) hot

b) cold

c) cool

d) warm

essential discoveries and accomplishments

In the space below, jot some notes about what concepts of this chapter were hardest for you to understand or remember. Imagine finding yourself suddenly in the role of "teacher" and consider what you would tell your "students" about these difficult concepts.

Share your *Essential Discoveries* with some of the other students in your class and ask if they are helpful to them. You may want to revise your notes based on good ideas shared by your peers. Under "Accomplishments," list at least three things you have accomplished since your last entry that relate to your career goals.

Discoveries:

_____

_____

_____

_____

_____

Accomplishments:

_____

_____

_____

_____

_____

Haircoloring

essential **objectives**

After studying this chapter and completing the Essential Companion *components, you should be able to:*

1. Identify the principles of color theory and relate them to haircolor.

2. Explain level and tone and their role in formulating haircolor.

3. List the four basic categories of haircolor, explain their chemical effect on the hair, and give examples of their use.

4. Explain the action of lighteners.

5. Demonstrate the application techniques for a) temporary colors, b) semipermanent colors, c) demipermanent colors, d) permanent colors, and e) lighteners.

6. Demonstrate special effects haircoloring techniques.

essential **haircoloring**

Will I ever get over my fear of haircolor and be able to formulate and apply it successfully in the salon?

Without a doubt! Haircoloring is an art and you have just begun your training as an artist. This chapter is designed to help you begin to build your confidence with haircoloring in a practical and understandable way. Haircolor is considered to be the "cosmetic for the hair" in today's market. Your clientele are no longer afraid of haircolor, and your haircolor clientele will range from young teenage boys to grandmothers. You will learn that it is fun and easy and all your efforts will be rewarded financially in the salon.

essential **concepts**

"I know of no more encouraging fact than the unquestionable ability of man to elevate his life by conscious endeavor."
—Henry David Thoreau

What are the key concepts or elements in haircoloring that I need to know to be successful?

You will begin by learning about basic color theory, a refresher of what you learned in elementary school when you studied the colors of the rainbow. You will learn how to lighten dark hair to a light blond as well as how to darken lighter hair. You will learn about the reasons people color their hair and the psychological effects haircolor can have on an individual. You will learn about the Level System used by professionals and haircolor manufacturers to analyze the lightness or darkness of a color. As with any professional service, you will gain practice in performing a thorough client consultation prior to providing a haircolor service. Your haircolor training will take you from temporary haircolor through semipermanent, demipermanent, permanent, hair lightening and special effects haircoloring procedures.

essential experience

The Color Wheel

In the diagram below, place the colors that correspond with the color found on the wheel. You may use crayons, markers, colored pencils, watercolor paint, or actually cut the various colors out of magazines. Your goal is to depict primary, secondary, and tertiary colors and label each accordingly.

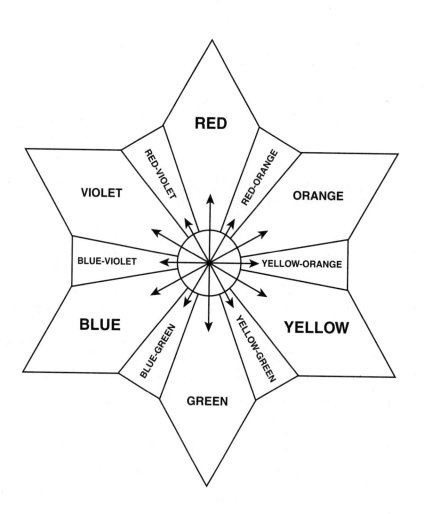

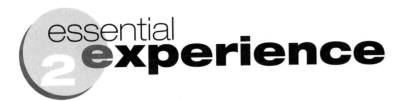

essential
2 experience

Haircolor Challenges

In the grid below, explain the solutions to the haircoloring challenges listed.

Challenge	Solution
Undesired Yellow Discoloration in Gray Hair	
Resistant Unpigmented Hair	
Damaged Hair Due to Blow-Drying, Harsh Products, Chemical Services	
Damaged, Overly Porous Hair	
Red Fading	
Brassiness	
Tint Back to Natural	

essential
3 experience

The Level System

Look through old magazines to find pictures of individuals that show the ten levels of hair or decolorization as stated in the chart below. Cut the colors out and paste them in the appropriate box in the chart.

Level 1 - Dark Red-Brown	**Level 2 - Red Brown**	**Level 3 - Red**
Level 4 - Red-Orange	**Level 5 - Orange**	**Level 6 - Orange-Gold**
Level 7 - Gold		**Level 8 - Yellow-Gold**
Level 9 - Yellow		**Level 10 - Pale Yellow**

essential
experience
4

The Four Classifications of Color

Haircolor is divided into four classifications: temporary, semipermanent, demipermanent, and permanent. The classifications indicate color fastness or the ability to remain on the hair. They are determined by the chemical composition and molecular weight of the pigments and dyes within the products found in each classification. Using the chart below, indicate the various characteristics of the four classifications of color. For molecular structure list the size and draw it in as well. Use external research as needed.

Classification	Temporary	Semipermanent/ Demipermanent	Permanent
Molecular Weight of the Dye Molecule			
Type of pH (acid or alkaline)			
Reaction or Change (physical and/or chemical)			
Color Fastness			
Color Effects (lifts/deposits)			

essential 5 experience

Windowpane—Color Applications

Windowpaning is the process of transferring key elements, points, or steps in a lesson into visual images that are hand sketched into the squares or "panes" of a matrix. Let your mind think in pictures and sketch the essential haircoloring concepts listed in each of the following windowpanes. Conduct additional research as applicable.

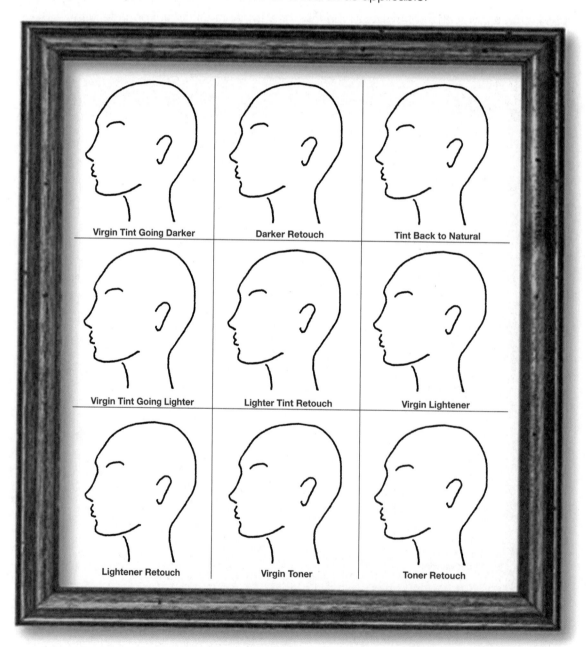

Virgin Tint Going Darker	Darker Retouch	Tint Back to Natural
Virgin Tint Going Lighter	Lighter Tint Retouch	Virgin Lightener
Lightener Retouch	Virgin Toner	Toner Retouch

essential
experience
6

Haircolor Crossword Puzzle

After identifying the appropriate word from the clues listed below, locate the word in the following crossword puzzle.

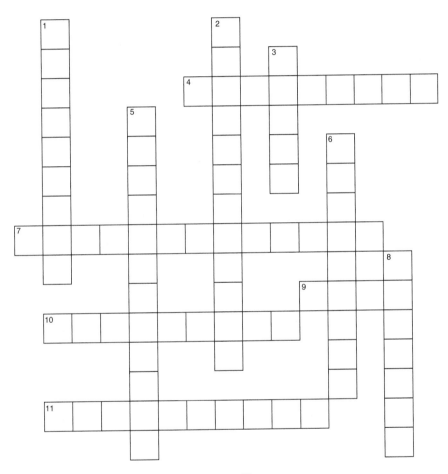

Across

4. Oxidizing agent that mixes with an oxidation color and supplies oxygen gas
7. Colors opposite each other on the color wheel
9. Technique involving slicing or weaving out sections
10. Chemical compound for decolorizing hair
11. Color left in hair after it goes through seven stages of lightening

Down

1. Oxidizer added to hydrogen peroxide to increase chemical action
2. Used to treat gray or resistant hair
3. Unit of measurement of lightness or darkness of a color
5. Coloring some strands lighter than natural color
6. Industry term referring to artificial haircolor products
8. 1/8" section of hair positioned over foil

essential
7 experience

Haircolor Word Search

After identifying the appropriate word from the clues listed below, locate the word in the following word search puzzle.

Word	Clue
_____	Hair painting
_____	Involves pulling hair through a perforated cap
_____	Used to ensure an even shade
_____	Coloring some strands lighter than natural color
_____	Strength of color tone
_____	Reverse highlighting
_____	Haircolor containing metal salts
_____	First step in double-process haircoloring
_____	Process of treating gray or resistant hair to allow better penetration
_____	Pure or fundamental color that cannot be achieved by mixing
_____	Color obtained from mixing equal parts of two primary colors
_____	Involves taking a 1/8" section of hair and placing it on foil
_____	Intermediate color achieved by mixing a secondary color with its neighboring primary color
_____	Permanent oxidizing color having the ability to lift and deposit in the same process
_____	Use primarily on prelightened hair to achieve pale or delicate colors
_____	The measure of potential oxidation of varying strengths of hydrogen peroxide
_____	Picking up strands with a zigzag motion of the comb

```
C  R  S  F  T  V  W  S  Y  V  F  J  K  V  H
A  C  E  L  G  L  C  N  A  Y  F  X  I  I  Y
P  R  E  L  I  G  H  T  E  N  I  N  G  N  N
T  R  M  C  L  C  Z  L  Q  G  F  H  T  J  N
E  O  E  P  E  I  I  Q  O  P  L  Q  K  J  M
C  B  T  S  T  B  F  N  R  I  Y  H  V  A  B
H  M  A  L  O  W  L  I  G  H  T  I  N  G  A
N  W  L  G  N  F  M  H  F  Q  I  R  F  Y  L
I  T  L  P  E  A  T  H  B  R  S  O  U  V  A
Q  N  I  P  R  I  S  E  C  O  N  D  A  R  Y
U  K  C  Y  N  E  M  G  N  V  E  A  S  R  A
E  T  O  G  G  U  Y  R  A  I  T  R  E  T  G
C  H  X  E  L  W  E  A  V  I  N  G  D  Z  E
G  I  V  O  I  A  P  A  U  P  I  G  O  C  E
L  L  V  P  N  I  G  N  O  H  T  N  C  D  T
```

essential experience

8

Haircolor Matching Exercise

Match each of the following essential terms with its definition.

_____ Analysis	
_____ Blonding	
_____ Coating	
_____ Degree	
_____ Enzyme	
_____ Keratin	
_____ Melanin	
_____ Overporosity	
_____ pH	
_____ Primary color	

1. The degree of acidity or alkalinity of any water solution.
2. An examination of the hair.
3. A term applied to lightening the hair.
4. Pigment that is fundamental and cannot be made.
5. The condition where hair reaches an undesirable stage of porosity.
6. Residue left on the outside of the hair shaft.
7. Granules scattered throughout the cortex like chips in a chocolate chip cookie.
8. The protein material in the hair.
9. A protein molecule that initiates a chemical process.
10. Various units of measurement.

essential
experience
9

The Client Consultation

In the space provided below, list all the steps required to complete a thorough haircolor consultation. Then choose another student as your partner. Conduct a haircolor client consultation on each other. Record your results on the school's client record card and standard consultation form.

1. _____
   _____

2. _____
   _____

3. _____
   _____

4. _____
   _____

5. _____
   _____

6. _____
   _____

7. _____
   _____

8. _____
   _____

9. _____
   _____

10. _____
    _____

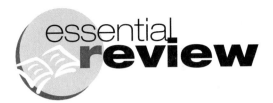
essential **review**

Complete the following review of Chapter 16, "Haircoloring," by circling the correct answer to each question.

1. _____ are specialized preparations designed to help equalize porosity and deposit a base color in one application.
   a) presofteners
   b) color conditioners
   c) conditioning activators
   d) fillers

2. A system for understanding the relationships of color is called _____.
   a) the law of color
   b) the Level System
   c) the color wheel
   d) primary color system

3. A _____ lightener is generally used for a lightener retouch because its consistency helps prevent overlapping of previously lightened hair.
   a) oil
   b) cream
   c) powder
   d) paste

4. A product prepared by combining permanent haircolor, hydrogen peroxide, and shampoo is _____.
   a) soap cap
   b) highlighting shampoo
   c) color filler
   d) highlighting shampoo tint

5. A mixture of shampoo and hydrogen peroxide creates a _____.
   a) soap cap
   b) highlighting shampoo
   c) color filler
   d) highlighting shampoo tint

6. A non-ammonia color that adds shine and tone to the hair is called a _____.
   a) polish
   b) wax
   c) spray
   d) glaze

7. A process that lightens and colors hair in a single application is known as _____.
   a) double-process haircoloring
   b) temporary rinsing
   c) single-process haircoloring
   d) virgin haircoloring

8. A patch test is generally conducted behind the ear or on the _____.
   a) inner wrist
   b) inner forearm
   c) temple or forehead
   d) inside of elbow

9. A combination of equal parts of prepared tint and shampoo that is applied to hair like regular shampoo is called a _____.
   a) color filler
   b) hair presoftener
   c) soap cap
   d) shampoo tint

10. A/an _____ is an oxidizing agent that, when mixed with an oxidative haircolor, supplies the necessary oxygen gas to develop color molecules and create a change in hair color.

a) activator

b) protinator

c) prohibitor

d) developer

11. After the hair goes through the ten stages of decolorizing, the color that is left in the hair is known as its _____ .

a) foundation

b) base

c) vertex

d) apex

12. An example of a natural or vegetable haircolor obtained from the leaves or bark of plants is _____ .

a) henna

b) tint

c) toner

d) demipermanent

13. Chemical compounds that lighten hair by dispersing, dissolving, and decolorizing the natural hair pigment are _____ .

a) dispersers

b) dissolvers

c) decolorizers

d) lighteners

14. Colored mouses and gels are considered to be what haircolor category?

a) permanent

b) semipermanent

c) demipermanent

d) temporary

15. Colors achieved by mixing equal parts of two primary colors are called _____ colors.

a) secondary

b) tertiary

c) neutral

d) protein

16. Colors with a predominance of red are considered to be _____ tones.

a) warm

b) cool

c) neutral

d) primary

17. Colors with a predominance of blue are considered to be _____ tones.

a) warm

b) cool

c) neutral

d) primary

18. Equal parts of blue and yellow mixed together create _____ .

a) pink

b) violet

c) green

d) orange

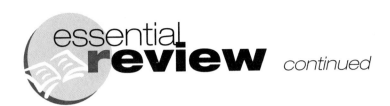

essential **review** *continued*

19. Equal parts of red and yellow mixed together create _____.

    a) pink   b) violet

    c) green   d) orange

20. Equal parts of red and blue mixed together create _____.

    a) pink   b) violet

    c) green   d) orange

21. Hair texture is determined by the _____ of the individual hair strand.

    a) length   b) strength

    c) diameter   d) color

22. Haircolor that is ideal for covering unpigmented hair, refreshing faded permanent color, depositing tonal changes without lift, corrective coloring, and reverse highlighting is

    _____.

    a) permanent   b) semipermanent

    c) demipermanent   d) temporary

23. Haircolor that is mixed with a developer and remains in the hair shaft until the new growth of hair occurs is called _____.

    a) permanent   b) semipermanent

    c) demipermanent   d) temporary

24. Haircoloring products fall into four categories including temporary, semipermanent,

    _____.

    a) permanent and perpetual   b) permanent and demipermanent

    c) demipermanent and perpetual   d) vegetable and demipermanent

25. Metallic haircolors are also called _____ colors.

    a) advancing   b) gradual

    c) delayed   d) accelerated

26. One safety precaution in haircoloring is to never apply tint if _____ are present.

    a) parents   b) children

    c) abrasions   d) dandruff particles

27. Permanent haircolor is applied by either the bowl-and-brush method or with a/an

    _____.

    a) spatula and brush   b) applicator bottle

    c) bowl-and-bottle   d) brush-and-bottle

essential review *continued*

28. Porous hair of the same color level will lighten faster than hair that is nonporous, because the bleaching agent can enter the _____ more rapidly.

a) medulla

b) cortex

c) cuticle

d) follicle

29. Primary and secondary colors that are positioned opposite each other on the color wheel are considered to be _____.

a) neutral

b) complementary

c) contradictory

d) contrary

30. Products created to remove artificial pigment from the hair are known as _____.

a) color or tint removers

b) pigment or melanin removers

c) porosity removers

d) highlight removers

31. The predominant tonality of an existing color is referred to as a _____.

a) base color

b) even color

c) neutral color

d) deep color

32. The cortex or middle layer of the hair gives strength and elasticity and contributes about _____ percent to the overall strength of the hair.

a) 10

b) 20

c) 60

d) 80

33. The strength of a color tone is referred to as _____.

a) level

b) value

c) depth

d) intensity

34. The measure of the potential oxidation of varying strengths of hydrogen peroxide is _____.

a) density

b) value

c) volume

d) percentage

35. The cuticle of the hair protects the interior and contributes _____ percent to the overall strength of the hair.

a) 10

b) 20

c) 60

d) 80

36. The U. S. Federal Food, Drug, and Cosmetic Act prescribes that a patch test, also called a/an _____ test, be given twenty-four to forty-eight hours prior to an application of aniline derivative tint.

a) predisposition

b) allergy

c) reaction

d) postdisposition

essential review *continued*

37. The term used to describe the warmth or coolness of a color is _____ .

a) mixed melanin

b) contributing pigment

c) tone or tonality

d) value or depth

38. The preliminary strand test will tell you how the hair will react to the color formula and indicate _____ .

a) application method

b) processing time

c) client satisfaction

d) application time

39. The method used to analyze the lightness or darkness of a hair color, whether natural or artificial, is called _____ .

a) the law of color

b) the Level System

c) the color wheel

d) primary color system

40. The tint formula in permanent haircolor contains uncolored dye _____ , which are small compounds that can diffuse into the hair shaft.

a) successors

b) precursors

c) activators

d) protinators

41. The melanin found in red hair is known as _____ .

a) pheomelanin

b) eumelanin

c) neomelanin

d) euromelanin

42. The melanin that gives black and brown color to hair is known as _____ .

a) pheomelanin

b) eumelanin

c) neomelanin

d) euromelanin

43. The ability of the hair to absorb moisture is called _____ .

a) density

b) texture

c) elasticity

d) porosity

44. The haircolor that partially penetrates the hair shaft and stains the cuticle layer, slowly fading with each shampoo, is known as _____ .

a) permanent

b) semipermanent

c) demipermanent

d) temporary

45. The number of hairs per square inch on the head relates to the hair's _____ .

a) density

b) texture

c) elasticity

d) porosity

essential **review** *continued*

46. The oxidizer that is added to hydrogen peroxide to increase its chemical action is known as the _____.

a) generator   b) penetrator

c) activator   d) accelerator

47. The technique of coloring strands of hair darker than the natural color is called reverse highlighting or _____.

a) foiling   b) frosting

c) lowlighting   d) streaking

48. The two methods of parting hair for a foil technique are _____.

a) slicing and striping   b) weaving and striping

c) slicing and threading   d) slicing and weaving

49. The free-form technique of hair painting is also called _____.

a) toning   b) balayage

c) brushing   d) swabbing

50. The first important guideline when color services do not turn out as planned or expected is _____.

a) call your instructor   b) apply color rinse

c) do not panic   d) give money back

51. The process of treating gray or very resistant hair to allow for better penetration of color is known as _____.

a) presoftening   b) prelightening

c) activating   d) accelerating

52. To some degree, the _____ is designed to protect the school or salon owner from responsibility for accidents or damages.

a) client record card   b) posted price list

c) release statement   d) indemnity insurance

53. What is added to hydrogen peroxide to increase its chemical action or lifting power?

a) accelerator   b) diffuser

c) dissolver   d) activator

54. What are the three types of hair lighteners?

a) oil, cream, powder   b) oil, paste, powder

c) cream, powder, paste   d) cream, paste, powder

essential review *continued*

55. What product is used to open the cuticle of the hair fiber so that tint can penetrate it?

   a) hair conditioner

   b) color filler

   c) alkalizing agent

   d) medicated shampoo

56. When performing retouches on red hair, the reds will last longer if you create them using a separate formula with a _____ haircolor product applied to the mid-shaft and ends of the strand.

   a) high-lift

   b) deposit-only

   c) temporary

   d) vegetable tint

57. When arranging for a haircolor service consultation, _____ walls are recommended.

   a) pastel-colored

   b) white or neutral

   c) bright-colored

   d) soft, yellow

58. When applying haircoloring products, always follow _____.

   a) manufacturer's directions

   b) your instincts

   c) client's directions

   d) personal preference

59. Which type of lightener is not used directly on the scalp?

   a) oil

   b) cream

   c) powder

   d) paste

60. Which type of haircolor product uses the largest pigment molecules?

   a) permanent

   b) semipermanent

   c) demipermanent

   d) temporary

essential
discoveries and accomplishments

In the space below, jot some notes about what concepts of this chapter were hardest for you to understand or remember. Imagine finding yourself suddenly in the role of "teacher" and consider what you would tell your "students" about these difficult concepts.

Share your *Essential Discoveries* with some of the other students in your class and ask if they are helpful to them. You may want to revise your notes based on good ideas shared by your peers. Under "Accomplishments," list at least three things you have accomplished since your last entry that relate to your career goals.

Discoveries:

_____

_____

_____

_____

_____

Accomplishments:

_____

_____

_____

_____

_____

_____

Histology of the Skin

essential **objectives**

After studying this chapter and completing the Essential Companion *components, you should be able to:*

1. Describe the structure and composition of the skin.

2. List the functions of the skin.

3. Describe the aging process and the factors that influence the aging of the skin.

4. Define important terms relating to skin disorders.

5. Discuss which skin disorders may be handled in the salon and which should be referred to a physician.

essential histology of the skin

Why do I need to learn about the skin and its disorders when I really want to specialize as a hair designer?

You actually do not need the level of knowledge that a scientist would have on this subject matter. However, a thorough knowledge of the underlying structures of the skin, nails, and hair will benefit you in your role as a professional cosmetologist. The skin is the largest and one of the most important organs of the body. Therefore, it becomes one of the most important subjects about which you need to know because so many cosmetology services deal directly with the skin—whether you are providing a hair and/or scalp service, a facial or skin care service, or a nail care service. All those services require you to come in direct contact with the client's skin. Knowledge of the skin will help you achieve the best possible results when providing hair, skin, and nail care services, while also providing the safest care for your client. Remember, happy clients come back and often bring their friends. That means more financial success for you.

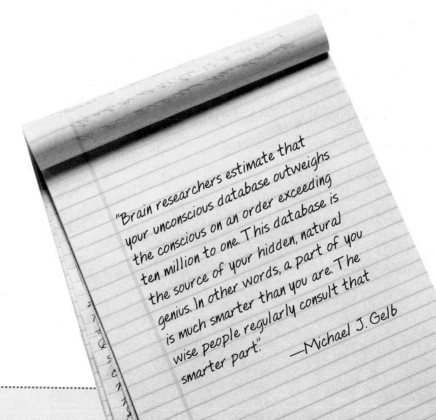

"Brain researchers estimate that your unconscious database outweighs the conscious on an order exceeding ten million to one. This database is the source of your hidden, natural genius. In other words, a part of you is much smarter than you are. The wise people regularly consult that smarter part."

—Michael J. Gelb

essential concepts

What do I need to know about the histology of the skin in order to perform professionally as a cosmetologist?

You need to become familiar with common disorders and diseases of the skin and recognize those conditions that cannot be treated or serviced by a cosmetologist. By thoroughly analyzing the functions, structure, and components of the skin, you will better understand how the skin actually works. You will learn that with proper care, your skin and the skin of your clients can remain young and look radiant for many years. You will need to understand how the skin is nourished and how the various glands affect the functions of the skin. You will need to recognize the many disorders the skin can experience and know how to treat them. The chapter also contains a significant number of new terms and definitions that will be meaningful to you in your career as a cosmetologist.

essential
1 experience

Analysis of the Epidermis

Using the chart below, analyze the structure of the epidermis. The first column lists each layer; in the second column, explain what quality this structure adds to the skin; and in the third column, list the purpose of the layer.

Layer	Composition	Purpose
Stratum corneum		
Stratum lucidum (clear layer)		
Stratum granulosum (granular layer)		
Stratum germinativum (basal or malpighian layer)		

essential
2 experience

Skin Layer Reconstruction

Using various household items or food products, create a model cross-section of the following layers of the skin:

Stratum corneum

Stratum lucidum

Stratum granulosum

Stratum germinativum

Papillary layer

Reticular layer

Subcutaneous

Either paste your items in the space provided or use poster board to make a larger model. (Hint: Items you might use include Rice Krispies, corn flakes, Fruit Loops, honey, a slice of bread, and/or a soft flour tortilla.) Once you've built your model, compare it to Figure 17-1 in your textbook.

essential
3 experience

Match each of the following essential functions of the skin with its description.

_____ Protection

_____ Sensation

_____ Heat regulation

_____ Excretion

_____ Secretion

_____ Absorption

1. Sebum or oil that lubricates the skin, keeping it soft and pliable. Oil also keeps hair soft. Emotional stress can increase the flow of sebum.

2. Perspiration from the sweat glands is eliminated through the skin. Water lost through perspiration takes salt and other chemicals with it.

3. The skin shields the body from injury and bacterial invasion. The outermost layer of the epidermis is covered with a thin layer of sebum, thus rendering it waterproof. It is resistant to wide variations in temperature, minor injuries, chemically active substances, and many forms of bacteria.

4. Through the nerve endings, the skin responds to heat, cold, touch, pressure, and pain. When nerve endings are stimulated, a message is sent to the brain that directs you to respond accordingly.

5. An ingredient or chemical can enter the body through the skin and influence it to a minor degree. Fatty materials, such as lanolin creams, are taken in largely through hair follicles and sebaceous gland openings.

6. The skin protects the body from the environment by maintaining a constant internal body temperature of about 98.6 degrees Fahrenheit. As changes occur in the outside temperature, the blood and sweat glands make necessary adjustments and the body is cooled by the evaporation of sweat.

essential
4 experience

Elasticity

Find a piece of fairly new elastic; stretch it to see how it easily reverts to its original shape. Then imagine a number of ways you can expose or abuse the elastic strip in much the same way the skin is abused. Perhaps you will place it in too hot a dryer, use harsh chemicals on it such as soaking it in bleach, constantly stretch it, and so on. Observe and record how after the elastic band has undergone certain exposure and abuse, it will no longer revert to its original shape. The same type of thing happens to our skin as we age. The more time we spend in the sun, the less we moisturize our skin, and so forth, the less elasticity it has.

_____

_____

_____

_____

_____

_____

_____

_____

_____

_____

essential
5 experience

Primary and Secondary Lesions

From the options listed below, label each of the primary and secondary lesions found in the drawing. After labeling them, write the definition of each type in the space provided.

Macule _____

Papule _____

Wheal _____

Tubercle _____

Tumor _____

Vesicle _____

Bulla _____

Pustule _____

Cyst _____

Scale _____

Crust _____

Excoriation _____

Fissure _____

Ulcer _____

Scar _____

Keloid _____

Stain _____

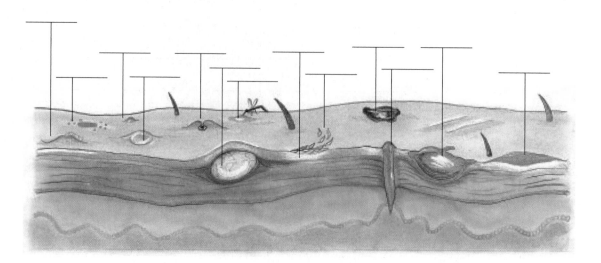

essential experience

Crossword Puzzle

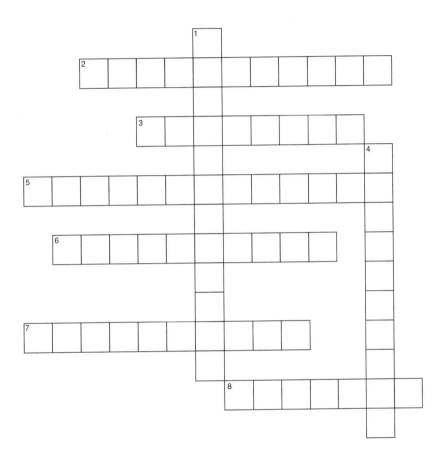

Across

2. Skin sore or abrasion from scratching or scraping
3. Blackhead
5. Excessive sweating
6. Deficiency in perspiration
7. Inflammatory skin condition
8. Protein that forms elastic tissue

Down

1. Foul-smelling perspiration
4. Dry, scaly skin caused by old age and exposure to cold

essential
experience
7

Crossword Puzzle

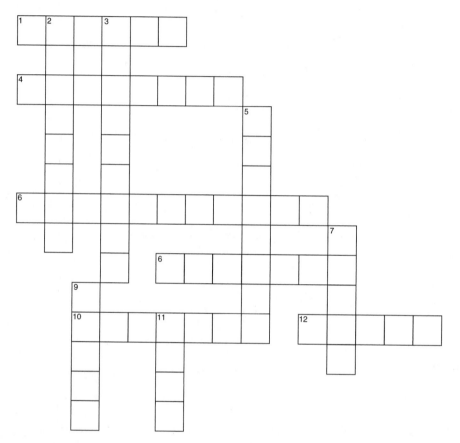

Across

1. Inflammatory, painful itching disease
4. Absence of melanin pigment
6. Study of skin
8. Crack in the skin
10. Chronic congestion on cheeks and nose
12. Large blister

Down

2. Protein giving skin form and strength
3. Outermost layer of skin
5. Increased skin pigmentation in spots
7. Malformation of skin due to abnormal pigmentation
9. Dead cells that form over a wound
11. Characterized by chronic inflammation of the sebaceous glands

essential experience

8

Word Search

Write the term for each definition below and then find them in the word search puzzle.

_____ Closed, abnormally developed sac, containing fluid, semifluid, or morbid matter, above or below the skin.

_____ Coiled base of sudoriferous (sweat) gland.

_____ Abnormal growth of the skin

_____ Skin disorder characterized by light abnormal patches.

_____ Small, brownish spot or blemish on the skin.

_____ Inflamed pimple containing pus.

_____ Skin condition caused by abnormal increase of secretion from the sebaceous glands.

_____ Abnormal brown or wine-colored skin discoloration with a circular and irregular shape.

_____ Sebaceous cyst or fatty tumor.

_____ Abnormal rounded, solid lump above, within, or under the skin; larger than a papule.

_____ An abnormal cell mass resulting from excessive multiplication of cells, varying in size, shape, and color.

_____ Open lesion on the skin or mucous membrane of the body, accompanied by pus and loss of skin depth.

_____ Technical term for wart; hypertrophy of the papillae and epidermis

_____ Milky-white spots (leukoderma) of the skin; acquired condition.

_____ Itchy, swollen lesion that lasts only a few hours; caused by a blow, an insect bite, urticaria, or the sting of nettle.

O	T	B	I	B	F	E	J	J	W	Y	T	B	k
E	O	E	D	F	Z	L	Y	T	H	E	L	G	E
F	G	Q	D	A	A	O	U	P	S	P	I	Q	M
G	E	D	J	E	M	M	O	Q	N	Y	L	L	I
Y	K	L	H	H	O	R	W	Q	D	G	C	X	L
P	K	W	C	R	T	X	E	Q	Z	W	F	V	C
U	I	Q	E	R	A	S	U	D	N	U	F	W	D
Y	X	Z	E	O	E	R	T	N	O	Y	N	C	M
P	U	P	I	B	T	B	E	A	G	K	D	F	O
U	Y	L	U	E	S	S	U	C	I	B	U	C	L
H	Y	O	H	S	L	U	N	T	L	N	D	E	O
D	P	U	J	C	T	V	E	E	I	U	G	Y	L
M	R	E	B	J	H	U	D	C	T	G	Z	T	I
K	I	J	Y	T	H	A	L	O	I	A	M	Y	W
Z	I	B	A	C	U	R	R	E	V	A	M	F	A

essential review

Complete the following review of Chapter 17 "Histology of the Skin," by circling the correct answer to each question.

1. The clear layer of the epidermis, consisting of small, transparent cells, is the _____.

   a) stratum lucidum   b) stratum granulosum

   c) stratum corneum   d) stratum germinativum

2. A skin sore or abrasion produced by scratching or scraping is a/an _____.

   a) excoriation   b) fissure

   c) ulcer   d) keloid

3. The basal or Malpighian layer, composed of several layers of different shaped cells, is also called the _____.

   a) stratum lucidum   b) stratum granulosum

   c) stratum corneum   d) stratum germinativum

4. The outermost layer of the skin is the _____.

   a) dermis   b) subcutaneous

   c) epidermis   d) adipose

5. The dermis is about _____ times thicker than the epidermis.

   a) 10   b) 25

   c) 35   d) 40

6. Which layer of the dermis houses the nerve endings that provide the body with the sense of touch?

   a) papillary   b) reticular

   c) corium   d) cutis

7. A condition of dry, scaly skin characterized by absolute or partial deficiency of sebum is _____.

   a) rosacea   b) asteatosis

   c) seborrhea   d) steatoma

8. The pliability of the skin depends on the elasticity of which skin layer?

   a) dermis   b) subcutaneous

   c) epidermis   d) adipose

9. The underlying or inner layer of the skin is the _____.

   a) dermis   b) subcutaneous

   c) epidermis   d) adipose

essential review *continued*

10. What is secreted by the sudoriferous glands?

    a) perspiration   b) blood

    c) odor   d) sebum

11. What controls the excretion of sweat?

    a) circulatory system   b) nervous system

    c) excretory system   d) respiratory system

12. A fatty layer found below the dermis is the _____.

    a) dermis   b) subcutaneous tissue

    c) epidermis   d) true skin

13. The skin responds to heat, cold, touch, pressure, and pain through stimulation of the _____.

    a) internal body temperature   b) sudoriferous glands

    c) sensory nerve endings   d) body fluid absorption

14. An itchy, swollen lesion that lasts only a few hours is a _____.

    a) wheal   b) tubercle

    c) bulla   d) macule

15. Wear a moisturizer or protective lotion with a sunscreen of at least SPF _____ on all areas of potential exposure.

    a) 10   b) 15

    c) 25   d) 30

16. No oil glands are found here.

    a) palms   b) face

    c) forehead   d) scalp

17. When checking existing moles for signs of cancer, look for asymmetry, differences in border, changes in diameter, and changes in _____.

    a) feel   b) smell

    c) color   d) symmetry

18. Smoking, drinking, taking drugs, and making poor dietary choices greatly influence the _____ process.

    a) developmental   b) stimulation

    c) sunscreen   d) aging

19. An abnormal rounded, solid lump above, within, or under the skin that is larger than a papule is known as a _____ .

    a) bulla   b) cyst

    c) pustule   d) tubercle

essential review *continued*

20. A thick scar resulting from excessive growth of fibrous tissue is a/an _____.

    a) excoriation   b) fissure

    c) ulcer   d) keloid

21. Another name for scar is _____.

    a) crust   b) excoriation

    c) ulcer   d) cicatrix

22. A skin condition caused by an excessive secretion of the sebaceous glands is _____.

    a) rosacea   b) asteatosis

    c) seborrhea   d) steatoma

23. A blister containing a watery fluid, similar to a vesicle but larger, is a _____.

    a) wheal   b) tubercle

    c) bulla   d) macula

24. A common, chronic, inflammatory skin disease whose cause is unknown is _____.

    a) eczema   b) psoriasis

    c) dermatitis   d) herpes simplex

25. Melanin protects the skin from the harmful action of _____.

    a) excessive heat   b) infrared rays

    c) pathogenic bacteria   d) ultraviolet rays

26. An acquired, superficial, round, thickened patch of epidermis due to pressure or friction on the hands and feet is a _____.

    a) mole   b) freckle

    c) keratoma   d) verruca

27. Another name for whiteheads is _____.

    a) milia   b) blackheads

    c) pimples   d) ulcers

28. An acute inflammatory disorder of the sweat glands, characterized by the eruption of small red vesicles and accompanied by burning, itching skin, is known as _____.

    a) steatoma   b) miliaria rubra

    c) hyperhidrosis   d) anhidrosis

29. A term used to indicate an inflammatory condition of the skin is _____.

    a) eczema   b) psoriasis

    c) dermatitis   d) rosacea

essential **review** *continued*

30. An abnormal growth of the skin is called _____.

a) hypertrophy

b) hypertrichosis

c) keratoma

d) callus

31. Vitamin _____ is an antioxidant that can help prevent certain types of cancers and has been shown to improve the skin's elasticity and thickness.

a) A

b) B

c) C

d) D

32. The best source for vitamin _____ is sunlight.

a) A

b) B

c) C

d) D

33. Drinking pure water sustains the health of the cells, aids in the elimination of toxins and waste, helps regulate body temperature, and aids in proper _____.

a) osmosis

b) metabolism

c) digestion

d) congestion

essential
discoveries and
accomplishments

In the space below, jot some notes about what concepts of this chapter were hardest for you to understand or remember. Imagine finding yourself suddenly in the role of "teacher" and consider what you would tell your "students" about these difficult concepts.

Share your *Essential Discoveries* with some of the other students in your class and ask if they are helpful to them. You may want to revise your notes based on good ideas shared by your peers. Under "Accomplishments," list at least three things you have accomplished since your last entry that relate to your career goals.

Discoveries:

_____

_____

_____

_____

_____

Accomplishments:

_____

_____

_____

_____

_____

Hair Removal

essential objectives

After studying this chapter and completing the Essential Companion *components, you should be able to:*

1. Describe the elements of a client consultation for hair removal.

2. Name the conditions that contraindicate hair removal in the salon.

3. List the two main classifications of hair removal and give examples of each.

4. Identify and describe three methods of permanent hair removal.

5. Demonstrate the techniques involved in temporary hair removal.

6. List the safety and sanitation precautions for hair removal.

essential hair removal

Why do I need to learn about removing unwanted hair when I may never provide such a service?

The technical terms for superfluous hair are *hirsuties* (hur-SOO-shee-eez) and *hypertrichosis* (hy-pur-trih-KOH-sis). Actually, the terms mean nothing more than hair growth occurring in unusual amounts or locations on either male and female clients. Often, those clients would like to have the hair removed, and that's where the professional cosmetologist comes in. History documents that everything from abrasive pumice stones to sharpened stones and seashells have been used to rub off and pluck out hair. Records also indicate that the Egyptians made a compound of mud and alum for this purpose, and the Turks used a combination of yellow sulfide of arsenic, quicklime, and rose water, which created a primitive depilatory called rusma.

At some point nearly every client will encounter unwanted hair in one area or another. In fact, excessive hair can be extremely embarrassing and unattractive for female clients, especially when the hair is found on the face and chest. It is essential that you master the techniques used for removal of unwanted hair, and also learn to be sensitive when approaching a client about this type of service.

essential concepts of hair removal

What do I need to know about hair removal in order to provide a quality service?

Hair removal falls into two major types: permanent and temporary. Salon techniques are generally limited to temporary methods. Permanent methods of hair removal include electrolysis (which is performed by a licensed electrologist), photo-epilation, and laser hair removal. Laws regarding photo-epilation and laser hair removal services vary in different states and provinces. However, the licensed cosmetologist should become proficient in all methods of temporary hair removal including shaving (if allowed in your state or province), tweezing, using depilatories, and a variety of epilation techniques.

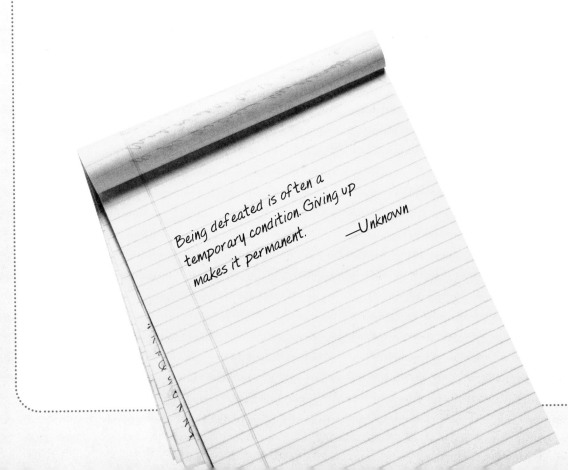

Being defeated is often a temporary condition. Giving up makes it permanent.

—Unknown

essential
experience
1

Temporary and Permanent Methods of Hair Removal

In the space provided, identify the following methods of hair removal as either permanent or temporary.

Hot wax _____

Shaving _____

Electrolysis _____

Tweezing _____

Electronic tweezing _____

Epilator _____

Cold wax _____

Photo-epilation _____

Laser _____

Depilatory _____

Threading _____

Sugaring _____

essential
2experience

Matching Exercise

Match the following essential terms with their identifying phrases or definition.

_____ Threading

_____ Cold wax

_____ Laser hair removal

_____ Tweezing

_____ Hot wax

_____ Electronic tweezing

_____ Epilator

_____ Shaving

_____ Sugaring

_____ Photo-epilation

1. Removes hair in large areas with a razor and cream.

2. Depilatory that can be used on the cheeks, chin, upper lip, nape, arms, and legs.

3. Procedure where a radio frequency transmits energy down the hair shaft into the follicle.

4. Used for clients who cannot tolerate heated wax.

5. A laser beam is pulsed on the skin, impairing the hair follicles.

6. Substance used to remove hair by pulling it out of the follicle.

7. The twisting and rolling of cotton thread along the skin surface, entwining the hair in the thread and lifting it from the follicle.

8. Commonly used for shaping the eyebrows.

9. Permanent hair removal treatment that uses intense light to destroy the hair follicles.

10. Temporary method of hair removal that uses a thick, sugar-based paste.

essential 3experience

Crossword Puzzle—Removing Unwanted Hair

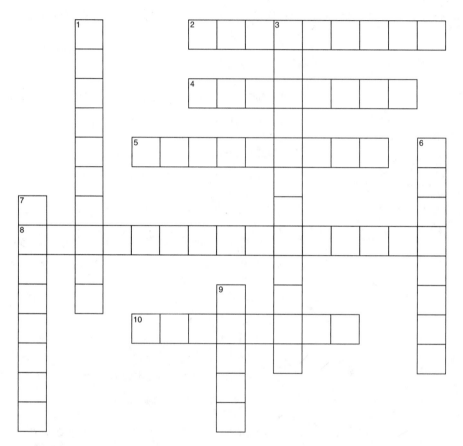

Across

2. Involves twisting and rolling cotton thread on the surface of the skin
4. Commonly used for shaping eyebrows
5. Excessive growth of hair
8. Permanent hair removal using intense light
10. Uses a thick, sugar-based paste

Down

1. Alkali substance for temporary hair removal
3. Hair removal by means of an electric current
6. Advisable to determine skin sensitivities
7. Substance used to remove hair by pulling from the follicle
9. A beam pulsed on the skin that impairs the hair follicle

essential
4 experience

Tweezing Eyebrows

Number the steps for an eyebrow tweezing procedure in the order in which they should occur.

Implements and Materials

_____ Antiseptic lotion, astringent

_____ Towels, tweezers, cotton balls

_____ Eyebrow brush, emollient cream

_____ Disposable gloves

_____ Gentle eye makeup remover

Preparation: Tweezing Eyebrows

_____ Wash and dry hands and put on disposable gloves.

_____ Recline client as for a facial. An alternative method is to seat client in a half-upright position and work from the side.

_____ Discuss the type of arch suitable for facial characteristics.

_____ Drape towel over client's chest.

Procedure

_____ Use mild antiseptic on cotton ball prior to tweezing.

_____ Cleanse eyelid area. Use cotton balls moistened with gentle eye makeup remover.

_____ Remove hairs from above the brow line. Brush hair downward. Shape upper section on one eyebrow; then the other. Frequently sponge the area with antiseptic.

_____ Brush eyebrows to remove powder or scaliness.

_____ Soften brows by saturating two cotton pledgets with warm water and place them over the brows for 1–2 minutes. Surrounding skin may be softened with emollient cream.

essential
experience
4

continued

_____ Remove hairs between brows by stretching the skin taut with index finger and thumb on nondominant hand. Grasp each hair individually with tweezers and pull with a quick motion in the direction of hair growth. Tweeze between brows and above brow line first. The area under the brow line is much more sensitive.

_____ Remove hairs from under the brow line. Brush hairs upward. Shape the lower section of one brow, then the other. Sponge the area with antiseptic.

_____ Sponge the tweezed area frequently with cotton moistened with an antiseptic lotion to avoid infection.

_____ Brush brow hair in its normal growth position.

_____ After tweezing, sponge brows and surrounding skin with astringent to contract the skin.

Cleanup and Sanitation

_____ Accompany client to reception area; suggest rebooking. Brows should be treated weekly.

_____ Continue makeup procedure if applicable.

_____ Remove towel and place in closed hamper.

_____ Wash hands with soap and warm water.

_____ Discard disposable materials in closed receptacle and disinfect implements.

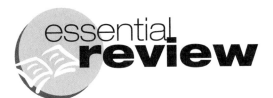

Using the words provided, fill in the blanks below to form a thorough review of Chapter 18, "Hair Removal." Words or terms may be used more than once or not at all.

abrasions	client procedure	hypertrichosis	radio frequency
acne	collagen	hypertrophy	energy
adhesives	depilatory	laser hair removal	rosacea
allergies	electrolysis	needles	rusma
aloe gel	emollient	normal	sensitive
anagen	epilator	opposite	shaving
beeswax	eyebrows	patch test	steamed
botox	hydroquinone	strand test	

1. Another technical term for hirsuties is _____.

2. A combination of yellow sulfide of arsenic, quicklime, and rose water that was used by the Turks as a crude hair removal agent is known as _____.

3. A client consultation prior to a hair removal service discloses all medications, both topical and oral, along with any known skin disorders or _____.

4. Facial waxing or tweezing should not be performed on clients who have _____ or very sensitive skin.

5. Recent _____ or collagen injections are considered to be a contraindication for facial waxing or tweezing.

6. Use of Retin-A, Renova, _____, or similar products contraindicates hair removal treatments.

7. Removal of hair by means of an electric current that destroys the root of the hair is known as _____.

8. Photo-epilation uses intense light to destroy hair follicles, has minimal side effects, and requires no _____.

9. A new method for the rapid, gentle removal of unwanted hair by means of a beam pulsed on the skin is called _____.

10. Laser hair removal is most effective when used on follicles in the active growing phase, or _____.

11. _____ is usually recommended for women when the unwanted hair covers a large area, such as the underarms and legs.

12. Correctly shaped _____ have a strong, positive impact on the overall attractiveness of the face.

13. Washing your hands thoroughly with soap and warm water is critical before and after every _____ you perform.

14. When tweezing the eyebrows, tweeze between the brows and above the brow line first because the area under the brow line is much more _____ .

15. The method that transmits _____ down the hair shaft into the hair follicle is called electronic tweezing.

16. Most manufacturers of electronic tweezers recommend that the area be _____ first in order to increase efficiency.

17. Depilatories contain detergents to strip the sebum from the hair and _____ to hold the chemicals to the hair shaft for the 5 to 10 minutes that are necessary to remove the hair.

18. If a client uses a chemical depilatory, you should perform a _____ to determine whether the individual is sensitive to the action of the product.

19. Wax is a commonly used _____ , applied in either hot or cold form as recommended by the manufacturer.

20. _____ has a relatively high incidence of allergic reaction.

21. When performing a wax service, the fabric strip and the wax that sticks to it is removed by pulling it in the direction _____ the hair growth.

22. Do not apply wax over warts, moles, _____ , or irritated or inflamed skin.

23. Apply _____ to calm and soothe sensitive skin that becomes red or swells due to a waxing procedure.

essential discoveries and accomplishments

In the space below, jot some notes about what concepts of this chapter were hardest for you to understand or remember. Imagine finding yourself suddenly in the role of "teacher" and consider what you would tell your "students" about these difficult concepts.

Share your *Essential Discoveries* with some of the other students in your class and ask if they are helpful to them. You may want to revise your notes based on good ideas shared by your peers. Under "Accomplishments," list at least three things you have accomplished since your last entry that relate to your career goals.

Discoveries:

_____

_____

_____

_____

_____

Accomplishments:

_____

_____

_____

_____

_____

Facials

After studying this chapter and completing the Essential
Companion *components, you should be able to:*

1. List and describe the five main categories of professional skin care products.

2. Explain the different skin types and skin conditions.

3. Identify the various types of massage movements and their physiological effects.

4. Have a general understanding of light therapy as it is used in facial treatments.

5. List and describe the different types of electrical currents used in facial treatments and the safety precautions that must be followed when working with them.

essential theory of massage

Why do I need to know about the underlying theory of massage, and are facials really that important in my career as a professional cosmetologist?

The term "massage" is of Arabic origin from the word *masa,* meaning to stroke or touch. The therapeutic benefits of massage were used and enjoyed in ancient Greece and are enjoyed more than ever today with the availability of licensed massage therapists. As a professional cosmetologist you will not only be given permission to invade the "comfort zones" of your clients, but you will be asked to actually touch them when you provide various services. For example, a good scalp massage can win the loyalty of your client for years to come. A massage that is both relaxing and stimulating accompanying a facial will inspire client confidence in you and will ensure repeat business. A firm massage given with flexible hands will ensure your clients receive the ultimate benefit from their services.

The generation born between the middle 1940s and the early 1960s is known as the baby boomer generation. As we enter the 21st century, that generation is growing older, ranging in age from their early 40s to their late 50s. With the aging of society, we have grown more interested in the health and beauty of the skin than ever before. Both men and women are buying more skin care products. The skin care industry is reported to be a multimillion-dollar-a-year business. Professional advice and professional services are essential in ensuring optimum results for those men and women who want to keep their skin looking healthy and youthful. That's where you, the professional cosmetologist, come in. With your knowledge and practiced skills, you can provide the services they desire while also increasing your annual income significantly.

Remember that no matter how the benefits of a service are stressed, unless it is enjoyable to the client, the need and demand for the service will decline. A facial service that is accompanied by a good massage will endear you to your clients for years to come. A satisfied client means more clients, and more satisfied clients means more income for you!

essential massage concepts

What do I need to know about the theory of massage and facials in order to provide quality services to my clients?

It is essential that you master the basic manipulations used in massage in order to ensure a satisfactory service as well as to eliminate harm or injury to your client. It will be helpful for you to understand the psychological effects that a good massage will have on your clients. You will master numerous massage manipulations and become familiar with the motor nerve points of the face and the neck.

As a licensed cosmetologist, you will be able to perform many services relating to skin care and makeup. Among those services will be facials, facial massage, packs, and masks. It should be ever present in your mind that you are about to become a professional in the image industry. Therefore, it is essential that you exemplify that role. In addition to learning how to provide the best possible services for your clients, you must be a role model for the industry you represent. You must have the most current hairstyle, the most well-manicured hands and nails, and the best cared for skin. Once you have developed all the applicable skills in this specialty area, you will be in high demand for employment in the high-end, full-service salons in your marketplace.

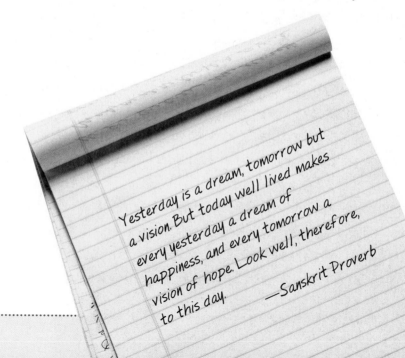

Yesterday is a dream, tomorrow but a vision. But today well lived makes every yesterday a dream of happiness, and every tomorrow a vision of hope. Look well, therefore, to this day.

—Sanskrit Proverb

essential **experience**

1

Motor Nerve Points

On the diagrams found below, identify the motor nerve points of the face and neck.

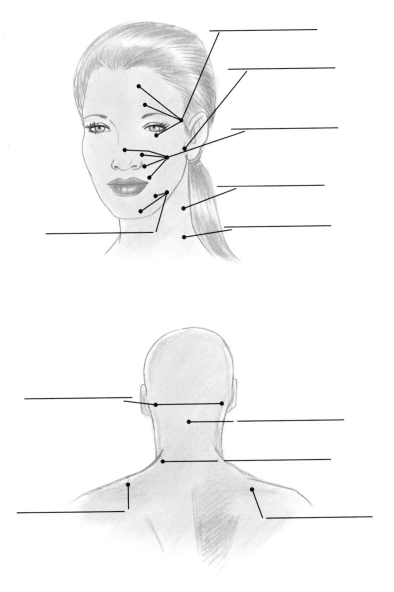

essential
2 experience

Match the following essential terms with their identifying phrases or definition.

_____ Effleurage	**1.** Tapping, slapping, and hacking movements.
_____ Petrissage	**2.** Light, continuous stroking movement.
_____ Friction	**3.** Shaking movement.
_____ Percussion	**4.** Kneading movement.
_____ Vibration	**5.** Restricted to the massage of the arm, hand, and foot.
_____ Joint	**6.** Deep rubbing movement.
_____ Rolling	**7.** Chopping movement performed with edges of hands.
_____ Chucking	**8.** Another term for percussion.
_____ Wringing	**9.** Pressing and twisting the tissues with a fast back-and-forth movement.
_____ Tapotement	
_____ Hacking	**10.** Grasping flesh firmly in one hand and moving the hand up and down along the bone while the other hand keeps the arm or leg in a steady position.
	11. Vigorous movement that applies a twisting motion against the bones in the opposite direction.

essential
3experience

The Elements of Massage Manipulations

Label each of the manipulations found below in the space provided.

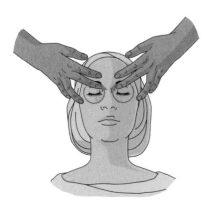

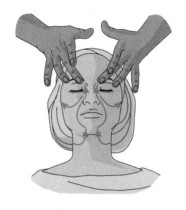

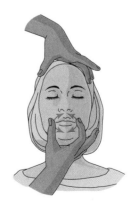

_____

_____

_____

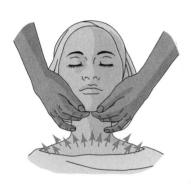

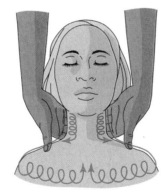

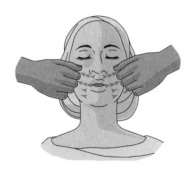

_____

_____

_____

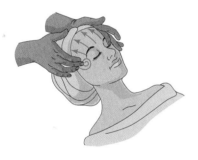

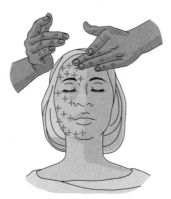

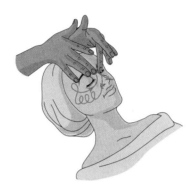

_____

_____

_____

essential
4 experience

Word Scramble

Scramble	Correct Word
agreleueff	_ _ _ _ _ _ _ _ _ _ *Clue:* Light, continuous stroking
atenotempt	_ _ _ _ _ _ _ _ _ _ *Clue:* Tapping, slapping, and hacking
cepnoirssu	_ _ _ _ _ _ _ _ _ _ *Clue:* Tapping, slapping, and hacking
gilnflu	_ _ _ _ _ _ _ *Clue:* Massaging the arms
gmasesa	_ _ _ _ _ _ _ *Clue:* Exercises facial muscles
inojt	_ _ _ _ _ *Clue:* Restricted to arm, hand, and foot
nbioitarv	_ _ _ _ _ _ _ _ _ *Clue:* Shaking movement
trmoo niopt	_ _ _ _ _ _ _ _ _ _ _ *Clue:* Each muscle and nerve has one
rcnfoiti	_ _ _ _ _ _ _ _ _ *Clue:* Deep rubbing movement
ragteissep	_ _ _ _ _ _ _ _ _ _ *Clue:* Kneading movement

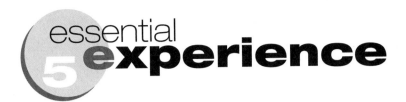

Massage Movements

In the chart below, describe each massage movement and list the parts of the body where the movement is used.

Name of Movement and Result Achieved	Movement Description	Where Used
Effleurage—		
Petrissage—		
Friction—		
Percussion—		
Vibration—		

essential
6 experience

Crossword Puzzle

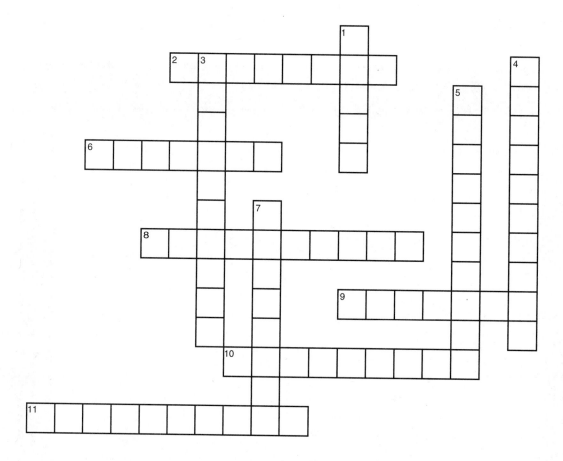

Across

2. A deep rubbing movement
6. Exercises facial muscles
8. Every muscle and nerve has one
9. A form of petrissage used mainly for massaging the arms
10. A shaking movement accomplished by rapid muscular contractions in your arm
11. A kneading movement

Down

1. Movements restricted to the massage of the arm, hand, and foot
3. Achieved through light but firm and slow rhythmic movements
4. Light, continuous stroking movement applied with the fingers
5. Tapotement
7. A vigorous movement in which your hands are placed a short distance apart

essential
7 experience

Word Scramble

Scramble	Correct Word
puekam atyr	_ _ _ _ _ _ _ _ _ _ _ _
nlaec thsee	_ _ _ _ _ _ _ _ _ _ _
laicaf eermtsa	_ _ _ _ _ _ _ _ _ _ _ _ _
askm	_ _ _ _
deah vocireng	_ _ _ _ _ _ _ _ _ _ _ _
eslwot	_ _ _ _ _ _
gsespno	_ _ _ _ _ _ _
ghhi qcyueerfn	_ _ _ _ _ _ _ _ _ _ _ _
itengtnrsa	_ _ _ _ _ _ _ _ _ _
fniredar mpal	_ _ _ _ _ _ _ _ _ _ _ _
gniclsnae mearc	_ _ _ _ _ _ _ _ _ _ _ _ _ _
ngifgniyam amlp	_ _ _ _ _ _ _ _ _ _ _ _ _
nolas wong	_ _ _ _ _ _ _ _ _
pslasuta	_ _ _ _ _ _ _ _
rirezuitsom	_ _ _ _ _ _ _ _ _ _
scpiitenat	_ _ _ _ _ _ _ _ _ _
irbultacgni ilo	_ _ _ _ _ _ _ _ _ _ _ _ _
siteus sptsri	_ _ _ _ _ _ _ _ _ _ _ _
rosabtneb tocnot	_ _ _ _ _ _ _ _ _ _ _ _ _ _ _ _
nottoc awssb	_ _ _ _ _ _ _ _ _ _ _ _
zuega	_ _ _ _ _

essential
experience
8

Mind mapping creates a free-flowing outline of material or information. Using the central or key point of preservative and corrective facials, diagram the purpose and benefits of such treatments. Use terms, pictures, and symbols as desired. Using color will increase retention of the material. Keep your mind open and uncluttered and don't worry about where a line or word should go as the organization of the map will usually take care of itself.

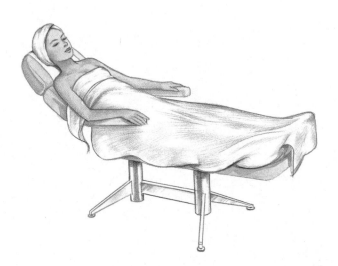

essential
9 experience

Client Consultation

Choose another student as your partner and conduct a facial treatment consultation on each other. Record your results on the sample record card found below. After the consultations, perform the appropriate facial service on each other. Ask an instructor to evaluate your procedure.

CONSULTATION CARD

Name _____   Date of Consultation _____

Address _____   D.O.B. _____

City _____ State ___ Zip _____   Occupation _____

Tel. (Home) _____ (Business) _____   Ref. by _____

Medical History   Contraindications

Current Medication _____

Previous treatments _____

Home Care Products used _____

SKIN TYPE   Oily   Normal   Dry   Combination

SKIN CONDITION   Clogged pores Sensitive Dehydrated Mature

Skin Abnormalities _____

Remarks _____

FACIAL RECORD

Date	Type of treatment	By	Products purchased

essential
10 experience

Crossword Puzzle

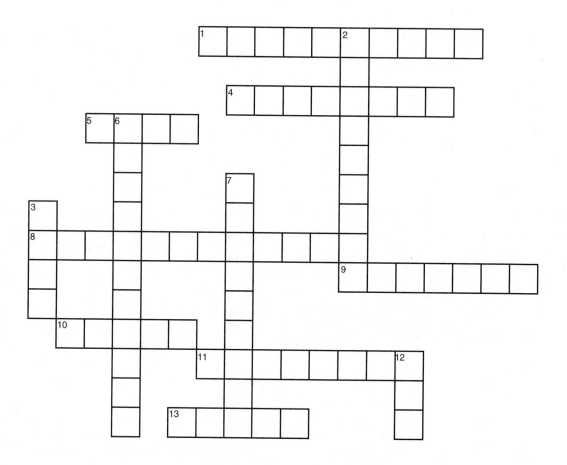

Across

1. Correcting facial skin conditions
4. Used to help soften superficial lines and increase blood circulation
5. A disorder of the sebaceous glands
8. Maintains the health of the skin
9. Used to remove the product from containers
10. Whiteheads
11. Lamp used in facial treatments
13. May be made from vegetables, fruits, dairy products, herbs, and/or oils

Down

2. Blackheads
3. Used to hold the towel in place
6. Gauze used to hold certain mask ingredients on the face
7. Covering used to protect the hair
12. Skin type caused by insufficient flow of sebum

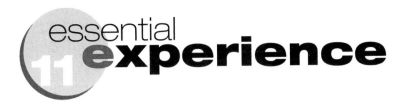

essential experience 11

Skin Care Product Research

Research a variety of skin care products available in your school and found at local supply stores. Include cleanser, toners, moisturizers, astringents, and so on. Use the chart below to track your findings.

Product Name	Pleasant Fragrance (Yes/No) Identify	Texture: How Does Product Feel?	Purpose of the Product	What Skin Type Is Product Used For?

essential
12 experience

Facial Steaming

Steaming the face can open pores, stimulate circulation, and help masks and creams work more effectively. Steaming should not be done more than once per week and should be accompanied by an appropriate moisturizer to avoid drying out the skin.

Try steaming at home by washing your face thoroughly and pinning or tying back your hair (or wear a shower cap). Boil a large pan of water and put in a handful of herbs based on your ingredient research. For example, chamomile, sage, peppermint, eucalyptus, and lavender disinfect and soothe the skin. They also contain oils that are beneficial to sinus passages. You can also use herbal oils from the health food store. Place the pan on a table or counter of appropriate height that will allow you to sit comfortably and hold your head over the pan. Lower your face over the pan and drape a large towel over your entire head and around the pan so no steam escapes. Now, relax and enjoy a highly rejuvenating experience. Steam for no more than 10 minutes. When finished, blot your face with a soft cloth. Your skin is now prepared for an effective exfoliation or mask treatment. If not continuing with these treatments, refresh the skin with cool water to close the pores. In the space provided, record the results, your skin's reaction, and how the procedure made you feel.

_____

_____

_____

_____

_____

_____

_____

_____

essential review

Using the following words, fill in the blanks below to form a thorough review of Chapter 19, "Facials." Words or terms may be used more than once or not at all.

3 to 5	effleurage	hands and arms	percussion
5 to 7	emollients	liquifying sebum	petrissage
7 to 10	enzyme peels	massage cream	preservative
alphahydroxy acids	essential oils	massage	relaxation
ampules	exfoliation	microdermabrasion	rolling
astringents	face wash	modelage	soft hands
clay masks	fresheners	moisturizers	sulfur
cleansing cream	from insertion to	motor	tonic lotion
cleansing lotion	origin	normal	tonic lotions
client consultation	fulling	oily	treatment
combination	gauze	open skin pores	vibration
dehydration	gommage	origin	warm, moist towels
dry	hacking movement	paraffin	wringing

1. _____ creams are used to hydrate and condition the skin during the night when normal tissue repair is taking place.

2. _____ can be used to hold in place certain mask ingredients that tend to run.

3. _____ is a vigorous movement in which your hands are placed a little distance apart on both sides of the client's arm or leg. While working downward, a twisting motion is applied against the bones in the opposite direction.

4. _____ is used to achieve good slip during a massage.

5. A water-based emulsion that can be used twice daily on normal and combination skin for the purpose of removing makeup and soil is known as _____.

6. A light-textured, oil-based emulsion used primarily to dissolve makeup and soil quickly is called _____.

7. A detergent-type foaming cleanser with a neutral or slightly acidic pH that varies in strength and texture is known as _____.

8. A light, continuous movement applied with fingers and palms in a slow, rhythmic manner without pressure is called _____.

essential review *continued*

9. A form of petrissage in which the tissue is grasped, gently lifted, and spread out is called _____.

10. A form of petrissage which is used mainly for massaging the arms is known as _____.

11. A shaking movement accomplished by rapid muscular contractions in the cosmetologist's arms, while the balls of the fingertips are pressed firmly on the point of application is known as _____.

12. Agents that soften or smooth the skin surface are called _____.

13. An enzyme peel in which a cream is applied to the skin before steaming and forms a hardened crust that is then massaged or "rolled" off the skin is called _____.

14. Another name for chemical exfoliation procedures is _____.

15. Aromatherapy refers to the therapeutic use of _____.

16. Clay preparations used to stimulate circulation and temporarily contract the pores of the skin are _____.

17. Cleansing cream is removed for the skin with tissues, moist cotton pads, facial sponges, or _____.

18. Cosmetology services are generally limited to the scalp, face, neck, shoulders, upper cheek, back, feet, lower legs, and _____.

19. Every muscle and nerve has a _____ point, which is the point over the muscle where pressure or stimulation will cause contraction of the muscle.

20. Fresheners, tonics, and astringents are all used to remove excess cleansers and residue left behind by face wash cleansers and are called _____.

21. Glass containers that contain intensive, highly concentrated extracts in a water or oil base are known as _____.

22. In addition to a firm, sure touch and strong, flexible hands, quality massage requires self-control and _____.

23. Infrared lamp exposure during or after facial manipulations is given for _____ minutes.

24. Maintaining the health of the facial skin by using correct cleansing methods, increasing circulation, relaxing the nerves, and activating the skin glands and metabolism through massage is known as _____ facial treatments.

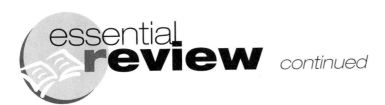

essential **review** *continued*

25. Masks that are melted at a little more than body temperature before application are
_____ masks.

26. Masks that contain special crystals of gypsum that harden when mixed with cold water
immediately before application are _____ masks.

27. Masks that have been found beneficial in reducing the production of sebum are
_____ masks.

28. One of the most recent advances in mechanical exfoliation is known as
_____.

29. Skin that may have either oily and normal areas or normal and dry areas is known as
_____.

30. Skin that is lacking in oil and often dehydrated is considered to be _____.

31. Skin that has an overabundance of sebum is considered to be _____.

32. Skin that is usually in good condition and has an adequate supply of sebum and moisture
is considered to be _____.

33. Steam the face mildly with warm, moist towels or with a facial steamer in order to
_____.

34. The fixed attachment of one end of the muscle to a bone or tissue is called the
_____ of muscles.

35. The most stimulating form of massage that is performed by tapping, slapping, or hacking
movements is called _____ or tapotement.

36. The type of tonic lotion with the lowest alcohol content which is beneficial for dry skin,
mature skin, and for sensitive skin conditions is _____.

37. The type of tonic lotion designed for use on oily or acne-prone skin is _____.

38. The product used for oily or acne-prone skin to loosen clogged pores in order to treat
and prevent the excessive buildup of dead cells that can cause acne lesions
is _____.

39. The manual or mechanical manipulation of the body by various movements to increase
metabolism and circulation, promote absorption, and relieve pain is _____.

40. The direction of massage movements should always be _____.

41. The result achieved through light but firm, slow rhythmic movements, or very slow, light
hand vibrations over the motor points for a short time, is _____.

42. The _____ movement involves pressing and twisting the tissues with a fast back-and-forth movement.

43. The condition that causes skin to feel dry and flaky because of an insufficient amount of water in the body is _____.

44. The first step of all facial treatments is the _____.

45. The term that refers to the peeling and shedding of the horny (outer) layer of skin is _____.

46. The product applied after the massage cream is removed is known as _____ or freshener.

47. The negative pole is the active electrode of the galvanic current when negative reactions are desired on the face, such as forcing negative ions into the skin, opening follicles, or _____.

48. Use of the wrists and outer edges of hands in fast, light, firm, flexible motions against the skin in alternate succession is called _____.

49. Water-based emulsions that are absorbed quickly without leaving any residue on the skin surface are called _____.

50. When the skin is grasped between the fingers and palms and tissues are lifted from the underlying structures and squeezed, rolled, or pinched with light, firm pressure, it is called _____.

essential discoveries and accomplishments

In the space below, jot some notes about what concepts of this chapter were hardest for you to understand or remember. Imagine finding yourself suddenly in the role of "teacher" and consider what you would tell your "students" about these difficult concepts.

Share your *Essential Discoveries* with some of the other students in your class and ask if they are helpful to them. You may want to revise your notes based on good ideas shared by your peers. Under "Accomplishments," list at least three things you have accomplished since your last entry that relate to your career goals.

Discoveries:

_____

_____

_____

_____

_____

Accomplishments:

_____

_____

_____

_____

_____

_____

Facial Makeup

essential objectives

After studying this chapter and completing the Essential Companion *components, you should be able to:*

1. List the types of cosmetics used for facial makeup and their purposes.

2. Describe correct makeup application procedures.

3. Identify the different facial types.

4. Demonstrate the different procedures for basic corrective makeup.

5. Demonstrate the application and removal of artificial eyelashes.

6. List the safety precautions to be observed in the application of makeup.

essential facial makeup

What makes applying makeup such a critical part of my career as a cosmetologist?

We've already discussed the fact that today's society is aging. As people age, they will do almost anything to feel and look younger. Makeup can do a great deal to emphasize attractive facial features and minimize those features that are not so attractive or are out of balance. Such an emphasis on attractiveness and makeup is not a new concept. History shows that both men and women, as far back as the New Stone Age, used tattooing and body paint for ornamentation. Makeup has been used for tribal identification, religious ceremonies, preparation for war (remember Mel Gibson in the movie *Braveheart*), and numerous other occasions and events. The Egyptians were quite innovative, using a combination of ground alabaster or starch mixed with vegetable dyes and mineral salts.

We have Elizabeth Arden and Max Factor to thank for making cosmetic makeup an industry of its own back in the 1930s. Without a doubt cosmetic makeup is here to stay. For a cosmetologist, that means more opportunity and more money!

essential concepts

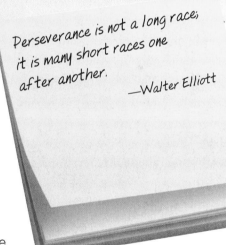

Perseverance is not a long race; it is many short races one after another.

—Walter Elliott

What do I need to know about facial makeup in order to provide a quality service?

In applying facial makeup, you need to consider the structure of the client's face, as well as the color of the eyes, skin, and hair. You also need to consider how the client wants to look, keeping in mind the reasonable results you will be able to achieve. For example, you can't change a large nose into a small, petite nose. You can, however, artistically and scientifically apply makeup and arrange hair so as to minimize the appearance of the size of the nose. You will truly become an artist when you can apply color, shading, and highlighting to create illusions that present the client in the most attractive manner. You will need to know all the techniques used for various face shapes and features. As a professional cosmetologist, you will be able to apply all those techniques combined with the appropriate hair color and design to create the best possible image for your client.

essential
experience
1

Commercial Cosmetics

Choose a partner and conduct a joint research project. Your goal is to create a collage of commercial cosmetics in at least two categories, such as daytime makeup, evening makeup, normal skin, dry skin, or oily skin.

Look through industry and fashion magazines and choose ads that depict various types of cosmetics such as lipstick, eye cream, moisturizer, foundation, mascara, and so on. Cut out the ads and use colored markers and other implements to create an artistic representation for your chosen category.

Your collage, built on a large poster board or other suitable background, should depict a complete cosmetic and skin care regimen for the category you have chosen. Be prepared to do an oral presentation to your classmates about your project explaining each product's purpose and how it is used.

essential experience

2

Windowpaning—Face Shapes

Windowpaning is the process of transferring key elements, points, or steps in a lesson into visual images that are hand sketched into the squares or "panes" of a matrix. Let your mind think in pictures and sketch the essential concepts printed in each of the following windowpanes. Don't be concerned with your artistic ability. Use lines and stick figures to depict the concepts requested.

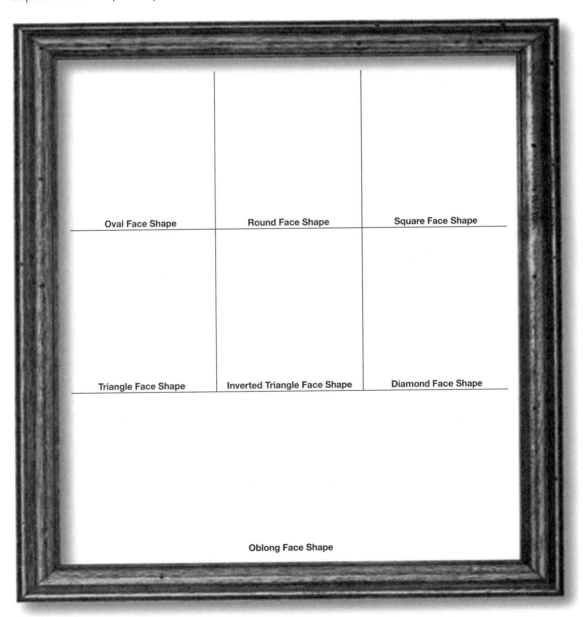

| Oval Face Shape | Round Face Shape | Square Face Shape |
| Triangle Face Shape | Inverted Triangle Face Shape | Diamond Face Shape |

Oblong Face Shape

essential
experience
3

Word Scramble

Scramble	Correct Word
ragel sone	_ _ _ _ _ _ _ _ _ _ _ *Clue:* Apply a darker foundation on the nose and a lighter foundation on the cheeks at the sides of the nose
talf seon	_ _ _ _ _ _ _ _ _ _ *Clue:* Apply a lighter foundation down the center of the nose, stopping at the tip
esolc tes seye	_ _ _ _ _ _ _ _ _ _ _ _ _ _ _ *Clue:* Apply shadow lightly up from the outer edge of the eyes
wanorr jnaliwe	_ _ _ _ _ _ _ _ _ _ _ _ _ _ _ _ *Clue:* Highlight by using a lighter shade foundation over the prominent area of the jawline
ayveh dilded	_ _ _ _ _ _ _ _ _ _ _ _ _ *Clue:* Shadow evenly and lightly across the lid from the edge of the eyelash line to the small crease in the eye socket
tsorh chtik nekc	_ _ _ _ _ _ _ _ _ _ _ _ _ _ _ _ _ *Clue:* Use a darker foundation on the neck than the one used on the face
doarb osen	_ _ _ _ _ _ _ _ _ _ _ *Clue:* Use a darker foundation on the side of the nose and - nostrils
wedi tes	_ _ _ _ _ _ _ _ _ *Clue:* Use the shadow on the upper, inner side of the eyelid
doabr wajenil	_ _ _ _ _ _ _ _ _ _ _ _ _ _ _ *Clue:* Apply a darker shade of foundation over the heavy area of the jaw, starting at the temples

essential experience 3 *continued*

Word Scramble (continued)

Scramble	Correct Word
ugnibgl yees	_ _ _ _ _ _ _ _ _ _ _ _ _ *Clue:* Minimize by blending the shadow carefully over the prominent part of the upper lid
gnol niht kcne	_ _ _ _ _ _ _ _ _ _ _ _ _ *Clue:* Apply a lighter shade foundation on the neck than the one used on the face
dnuor seye	_ _ _ _ _ _ _ _ _ _ *Clue:* Lengthen by extending the shadow beyond the outer corner of the eyes

essential
4 experience

Corrective Lip Treatment

Use colored pencils on the diagrams to illustrate how lipstick can be applied to create the illusion of more balanced and proportioned lips.

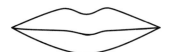

Thin lower lip

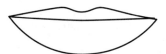

Thin upper lip

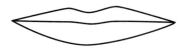

Thin lips

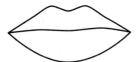

Small mouth

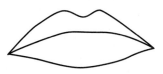

Drooping corners

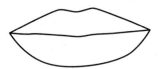

Oval lips

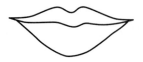

Sharp peaks

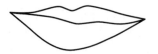

Uneven lips

essential 5 experience

Crossword Puzzle

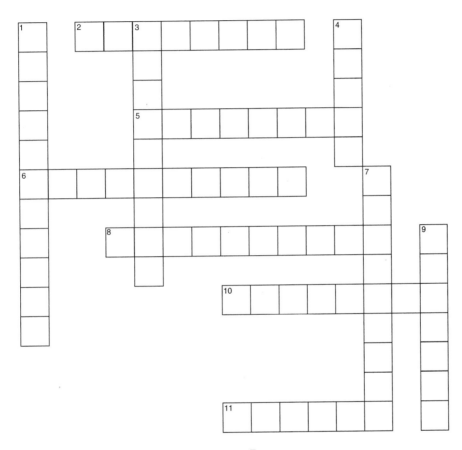

Across

2. Part of a complete and effective makeup application if well-groomed
5. Used to remove makeup from containers
6. Individual artificial eyelashes
8. Base or protective film
10. Used to remove excess facial hair
11. Used to add matte finish to face

Down

1. Used for theatrical purposes
3. Used to accentuate eyelids
4. Used to color cheeks
7. Used to cover blemishes
9. Used to darken, define, and thicken lashes

essential
experience
6

Band Lash Procedure

Number the following steps in the preparation, procedure, and cleanup activities for applying artificial band eyelashes in the order they should occur.

Preparation

_____ Wash your hands.

_____ Properly drape the client to protect her clothing and have her use a hairline strip, headband, or turban during the procedure.

_____ Gather and arrange the required implements, materials, and supplies.

_____ If the client has not already done so, remove all eye makeup so that the lash adhesive will adhere properly. Work carefully and gently. Follow the manufacturer's instructions carefully.

_____ If the client wears contact lenses, they must be removed before starting the procedure.

_____ Client consultation: Discuss with the client the desired length of the lashes and the effect she hopes to achieve.

_____ Place the client in the makeup chair with her head at a comfortable working height. The client's face should be well and evenly lit, but avoid shining the light directly into the eyes. Work from behind or to the side of the client. Avoid working directly in front of the client whenever possible.

Procedure

_____ Apply a thin strip of lash adhesive to the base of the lash and allow a few seconds for it to set.

_____ Brush the client's eyelashes to make sure they are clean and free of foreign matter, such as mascara particles. If the client's lashes are straight, they can be curled with an eyelash curler before you apply the artificial lashes.

_____ Carefully remove the eyelash band from the package.

essential
experience *continued*

6

_____ Feather the lash by nipping into it with the points of your scissors. This creates a more natural look.

_____ Apply the lower lash if desired. Lower lash application is optional, as it tends to look more unnatural. Trim the lash as necessary and apply adhesive in the same way you did for the upper lash. Place the lash on the top of the client's lower lash. Place the shorter lash toward the center of the eye and the longer lash toward the outer part of the lid.

_____ Start with the upper lash. If it is too long to fit the curve of the upper eyelid, trim the outside edge. Use your fingers to bend the lash into a horseshoe shape to make it more flexible so it fits the contour of the eyelid.

_____ Apply the lash. Start with the shorter part of the lash and place it on the inner corner of the eye, toward the nose. Position the rest of the artificial lash as close to the client's own lash as possible. Use the rounded end of a lash liner brush or tweezers to press the lash on. Be very careful and gentle when applying the lashes. If eyeliner is to be used, the line is usually drawn on the eyelid before the lash is applied and retouched when the artificial lash is in place.

Cleanup and Sanitation

_____ Sanitize your workstation.

_____ Wash your hands with soap and warm water.

_____ Disinfect implements such as eyelash curlers.

_____ Place towels, linens, and makeup cape in a hamper.

_____ Discard all disposable items, such as sponges, pads, spatulas, and applicators.

_____ Clean and sanitize brushes using a commercial brush sanitizer.

essential review

Using the following words, fill in the blanks below to form a thorough review of Chapter 20, "Facial Makeup." Words or terms may be used more than once or not at all.

antiseptic	double-dip	lip	powder foundation
blues	eye tabbing	lighter	smooth
complementary	eyeliner	matte	straight
concealers	feathering	misshapen	strip
contour	foundation	nose	thicker
contours	frame	paraffin	widening
cream	high arch	paste	yellow
discolorations	inner rim	pink	yellow or gold

1. Attaching individual eyelashes to a client's own lashes is referred to as _____.

2. A cosmetic, usually tinted, that is used as a base or as a protective film applied before powder is known as _____.

3. _____ foundations are predominantly water, mineral oil, stearic acid, cetyl alcohol, propylene glycol, triethanolamine, lanoline derivatives, borax, and insoluble pigments.

4. A powder base mixed with a coloring agent or pigment and perfume is known as a _____.

5. _____ are available in pots, pencils, wands, and tubes/sticks in a range of colors to coordinate with or match natural skin tones.

6. Face powder improves the overall attractiveness of the skin by enhancing the skin's natural color, helping to conceal minor blemishes and _____, and toning down excessive color and shine.

7. Cheek color gives a natural-looking glow to the face and also helps to create more attractive facial _____.

8. When applying cheek color, do not apply the color in toward the _____ beyond the center of the eye.

9. Lip color is a cosmetic in _____ form, usually in a metal or plastic tube, manufactured in a wide range of colors.

essential review *continued*

10. In addition to outlining the lips, lip liner helps to keep lip color from _____.

11. Eye shadows are applied on the eyelids to accentuate or contour them and come in a variety of finishes including metallic, _____, frost, shimmer, and dewy.

12. A highlight color is _____ than the client's skin tone and may have any finish including matte or iridescent.

13. A _____ color is deeper and darker than the client's skin tone and is applied to minimize a specific area to create contour.

14. The cosmetic used to outline and emphasize the eyes is called _____.

15. Eyeliner pencils consist of a _____ wax or hardened oil base with a variety of additives to create color.

16. According to the American Medical Association, eye pencils should not be used to color the _____ of the eyes.

17. Eyebrow pencils or shadows are used to darken eyebrows, to fill in sparse areas, or to correct _____ brows.

18. Mascara is used to enhance the natural lashes by making them appear _____ and longer.

19. Warm colors are dominated by _____ tones.

20. Cool colors suggest coolness and are dominated by _____.

21. When choosing eye makeup colors, consider contrasting eye color with _____ colors to emphasize the eye color most effectively.

22. When choosing makeup colors, take care to coordinate cheek and _____ colors within the same color family.

23. Concealer is applied before a _____.

24. When applying mascara to a client, use a disposable mascara wand and dip into a clean tube of mascara, taking care to never _____.

25. Properly reshaping and defining the eyebrows is essential to the best look for the client because the eyebrow is the _____ for the eye.

26. If eyes are close-set, they can be made to appear farther apart by _____ the distance between the eyebrows and extending them outward slightly.

27. When arching brows for a long face, making them almost _____ can create the illusion of a shorter face.

28. A square face will appear more oval if there is a _____ on the ends of the eyebrows.

essential
review *continued*

29. For ruddy skin, apply a _____ or green foundation to affected areas, blending carefully.

30. For sallow skin, apply a _____ or violet-based foundation on the affected areas and blend carefully into the jaw and neck.

31. Band lashes are also called _____ lashes.

32. As a safety precaution when giving a facial, keep fingernails _____ and avoid scratching the client's skin.

33. In order to avoid infection when arching eyebrows, use an _____ on the tweezed area.

essential discoveries and accomplishments

In the space below, jot some notes about what concepts of this chapter were hardest for you to understand or remember. Imagine finding yourself suddenly in the role of "teacher" and consider what you would tell your "students" about these difficult concepts.

Share your **Essential Discoveries** with some of the other students in your class and ask if they are helpful to them. You may want to revise your notes based on good ideas shared by your peers. Under "Accomplishments," list at least three things you have accomplished since your last entry that relate to your career goals.

Discoveries:

_____

_____

_____

_____

Accomplishments:

_____

_____

_____

_____

Nail Structure and Growth

essential objectives

After studying this chapter and completing the Essential Companion *components, you should be able to:*

1. Describe the structure and composition of nails.

2. Discuss how nails grow.

3. List and describe the various disorders and irregularities of nails.

4. Recognize diseases of the nails that should not be treated in the salon.

essential nails and their disorders

I am going to be a cosmetologist, not a scientist or doctor.
Why do I need to learn about nail diseases and disorders?

That's a very good question. The fact is that nail disorders and diseases are certainly not the most glamorous aspect of your training in cosmetology, but could be one of the most essential. More infections are spread through the nails and hands than any other area of the body. You actually have a greater chance of contracting a nail disease from a client than a skin disease or head lice. Therefore, careful analysis of the client's hands and nails is essential to both your safety and that of your clients. Think about it. If you contract an infection, it may prevent you from working for an extended period of time and that will cost you money, both in lost income and in medical expenses. So learning about the structure and growth of the nail and the diseases and disorders associated with the nails is extremely relevant to your future success and well-being.

essential concepts

Realize that true happiness lies within you. Waste no time and effort searchng for peace and contentment and joy in the world outside. Remember that there is no happiness in having or getting, but only in giving. Reach out. Share. Smile. Hug. Happiness is a perfume you cannot pour on others without getting a few drops on yourself.

—Og Mandino

What do I need to know about the nail, its structure, its growth, and its disorders in order to provide quality manicuring and pedicuring services?

You need to recognize that the condition of the nails may actually reflect the general health of the whole body. You need to understand the structure of the nail, as well as the structures surrounding the nail. Once you understand how nails grow, you will be better equipped to recognize the malformations, disorders, and irregularities that your clients may bring to the salon. You will need to be able to discern between disorders and infectious diseases that must be referred to a physician for treatment. When you've gained that knowledge, you can proceed confidently with appropriate nail services, knowing that you and your clients are not at risk.

essential
experience
1

Nail Diagrams

Label the parts of the nail on the front view and cross-section diagrams using the terms listed below. Note that some essential terms may be used more than once.

bone	lunula
cuticle	matrix bed (nail root)
eponychium	nail bed
free edge	nail body
hyponychium	nail plate

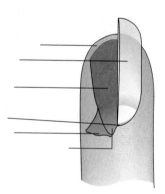

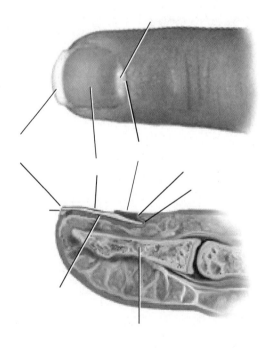

essential
2 experience

Match each of the following essential terms with its definition.

_____ Cuticle

_____ Eponychium

_____ Hyponychium

_____ Mantle

_____ Nail grooves

_____ Nail walls

_____ Perionychium

1. Slits or tracks at either side of the nail, upon which the nail moves as it grows.

2. The crescent of toughened skin around the base of the nails.

3. The thickened stratum corneum of the epidermis that lies underneath the free edge.

4. The portion of the epidermis surrounding the entire nail border.

5. Folds of skin overlapping the sides of the nail.

6. The extension of the cuticle at the base of the nail body that partly overlaps the lunula.

7. The deep fold of skin where the nail root is located.

essential

experience

3

Windowpane

Windowpaning is the process of transferring key elements, points, or steps in a lesson into visual images that are hand sketched into the squares or "panes" of a matrix. Let your mind think in pictures and sketch the essential concepts printed in each of the following window panes. Don't be concerned with your artistic ability. Use lines and stick figures to depict the concepts requested for the various shapes of the nail.

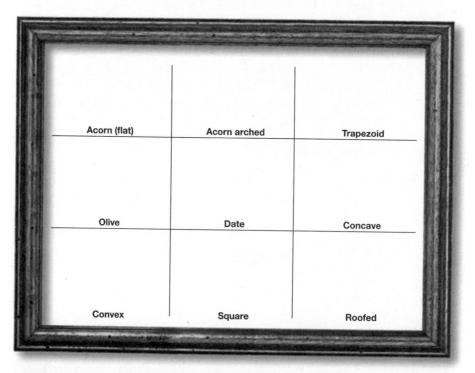

Acorn (flat)	Acorn arched	Trapezoid
Olive	Date	Concave
Convex	Square	Roofed

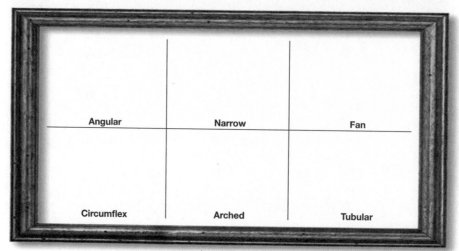

| Angular | Narrow | Fan |
| Circumflex | Arched | Tubular |

essential
4 experience

Nail Disorders, Irregularities, and Diseases

Label each of the following pictures or illustrations using the terms found below. Use your standard textbook and other references in the school's library to assist you.

Eggshell nail	Onychogryposis	Pyogenic granuloma
Furrows	Onycholysis	Tile-shaped nails
Hangnail	Onychomadesis	Tinea
Leukonychia	Onychophagy	Tinea pedis
Melanonychia	Onychorrhexis	Tinea unguium
Onychatrophia or atrophy	Paronychia	Trumpet or pincer nails
Onychauxis	Plicatured nail	
Onychocryptosis	Pterygium	

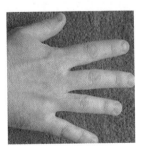
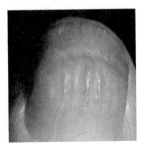
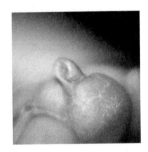
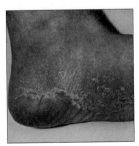

_____ _____

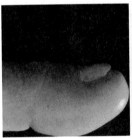
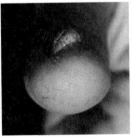
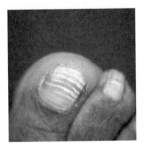
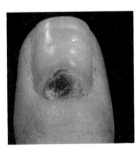

_____ _____

essential
experience
4
continued

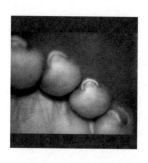

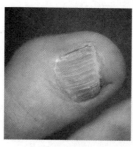

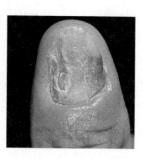

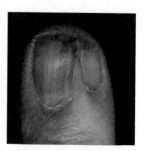

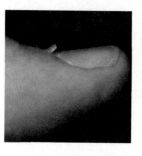

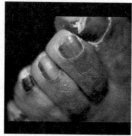

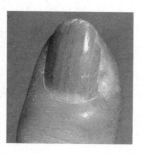

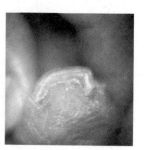

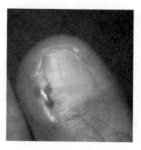

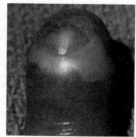

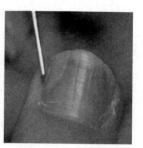

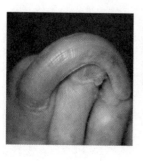

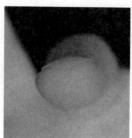

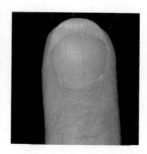

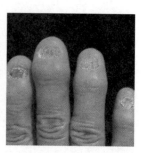

essential 5 experience

Match each of the following essential terms with its definition.

_____ Corrugation	**1.** Bitten nails
_____ Furrows	**2.** Hangnail or split cuticle
_____ Leukonychia	**3.** Overgrowth of nails
_____ Onychauxis	**4.** Wavy ridges
_____ Onychatrophia	**5.** White spots
_____ Pterygium	**6.** Horny growth of nail bed
_____ Onychophagy	**7.** Lengthwise or crosswise depressions
_____ Onychorrhexis	**8.** Noticeably thin, white nail plate more flexible than normal nails
_____ Agnail	**9.** Any deformity or disease of the nails
_____ Eggshell	**10.** Infectious or inflammatory condition of surrounding tissues
_____ Onychosis	**11.** Increased curvature; also called "ram's horn nail"
_____ Tinea	**12.** Ingrown nails
_____ Paronychia	**13.** Severe inflammation of the nail in which a lump of red tissue grows up from nail bed to nail plate.
_____ Onychia	**14.** Forward growth of cuticle
_____ Onychocryptosis	**15.** Periodic shedding
_____ Onychoptosis	**16.** Inflammation of matrix with formation of pus and shedding of the nail.
_____ Onycholysis	**17.** Atrophy or wasting away
_____ Pyogenic granuloma	**18.** Abnormal brittleness with striations
_____ Onychophosis	**19.** Ringworm
_____ Onychogryposis	**20.** Loosening of the nail without shedding

essential
experience
6

Word Search—Nail Structure

After identifying the appropriate word from the clues listed below, locate the word in the following word search puzzle.

Word	Clue
_____	Ringworm of the foot
_____	Dark purplish spots due to injury
_____	Wavy ridges
_____	The overlapping skin around the nail
_____	Thin, white nail plate which is more flexible than normal nails
_____	General term for vegetable parasites
_____	White spots in the nail
_____	Atrophy or wasting away of the nail
_____	Hypertrophy
_____	An inflammation of the nail matrix, accompanied by pus
_____	Ingrown nails
_____	Pertains to enlarged and increased curvature of the nail
_____	Bitten nails

```
S  I  S  O  T  P  Y  R  C  O  H  C  Y  N  O
N  K  U  R  O  N  Y  C  H  A  U  X  I  S  N
O  N  Y  C  O  P  H  A  G  Y  O  M  X  U  Y
I  G  N  U  F  M  Q  C  E  T  O  V  W  R  C
T  E  G  G  S  H  E  L  L  N  A  I  L  S  H
A  U  G  F  '  O  C  L  G  P  I  N  A  D  A
G  J  S  C  E  I  U  F  A  U  H  F  L  C  T
U  A  S  L  T  H  T  J  W  E  C  C  N  N  R
R  E  D  U  E  B  J  T  Q  L  Y  G  L  B  O
R  L  C  N  L  N  X  R  M  V  N  G  Y  B  P
O  N  Y  C  H  O  G  R  Y  P  O  S  I  S  H
C  Y  X  A  T  U  V  L  O  C  K  B  F  D  I
R  W  L  I  A  N  D  E  S  I  U  R  B  U  A
P  A  F  Q  K  U  P  J  E  I  E  E  O  I  V
W  S  Z  H  A  H  L  H  G  U  L  T  F  F  C
```

essential experience 7

Word Search—Nail Structure 2

After identifying the appropriate word from the clues listed below, locate the word in the following word search puzzle.

Word	Clue
_____	Extension of the cuticle at the base of the nail body that partly overlaps the lunula
_____	Another term for onychauxis
_____	Thickened stratum corneum of the epidermis that lies beneath the free edge of the nail
_____	Half moon
_____	Darkening of the fingernails or toenails
_____	Atrophy or wasting away of the nail
_____	The loosening of the nail without shedding
_____	Refers to a growth of horny epithelium in the nail bed
_____	Split or brittle nails
_____	An infectious and inflammatory condition of the tissues surrounding the nails
_____	Forward growth of the eponychium (cuticle)
_____	Ringworm

```
E  U  F  X  K  P  G  R  N  V  O  Q  A  M  A
O  N  Y  C  H  O  R  R  H  E  X  I  S  P  T
D  G  P  E  R  I  O  N  Y  C  H  I  U  M  E
L  N  S  S  Q  P  X  N  R  P  O  Y  X  O  P
V  Q  A  I  H  C  Y  N  O  N  A  L  E  M  O
F  O  L  I  S  D  V  R  Y  W  X  L  C  A  N
F  V  U  A  X  O  T  C  V  X  M  G  I  I  Y
S  S  N  O  F  A  H  L  S  I  X  H  N  S  C
Y  Y  U  L  H  O  W  P  W  O  C  J  Z  H  H
H  Y  L  C  L  S  T  I  O  Y  K  B  U  B  I
R  I  Y  Y  C  C  G  I  N  H  X  I  J  R  U
Y  N  S  Q  H  Y  P  O  N  Y  C  H  I  U  M
O  I  Y  H  P  O  R  T  R  E  P  Y  H  O  X
S  B  G  E  O  A  P  L  F  D  A  E  N  V  X
R  I  N  A  P  T  E  R  Y  G  I  U  M  O  N
```

essential
8 experience

Technical Term Mnemonics

Mnemonics are aids that can be used to assist your memory. They can be words or phrase associations, songs, or any other method that will trigger your memory of key terms or information contained in a lesson. For example, if you were trying to remember the three primary areas of haircutting, **b**lunt, **g**raduated, and **l**ayered, you might make up a sentence using the first letter of each type of haircutting. In this case, the mnemonic might be **B**renda **G**ot **L**ost. Using this learning tool, try to develop a mnemonic for each of the following technical terms in the study of the nail. For example: Ony**chop**tosis is the periodic shedding or falling off of the nail. Within the technical term is the word *chop*. You might relate the word *chop* to the chopping off or falling off of the nail and remember the meaning of onychoptosis. Give it a try with the other terms. Don't limit yourself to words. You can draw pictures or visualize circumstances that will prompt you to remember the technical term.

1. Corrugations _____
   _____

2. Furrows _____
   _____

3. Leukonychia _____
   _____

4. Onychomadesis _____
   _____

5. Onychauxis _____
   _____

6. Onychatrophia _____
   _____

7. Pterygium _____
   _____

8. Onychophagy _____
   _____

9. Onychorrhexis _____
   _____

10. Onychomycosis _____
    _____

11. Paronychia _____
    _____

12. Onychia _____
    _____

13. Onychocryptosis _____
    _____

14. Onychoptosis _____
    _____

15. Onycholysis _____
    _____

16. Pyogenic granuloma _____
    _____

17. Onychophosis _____
    _____

18. Onychogryposis _____
    _____

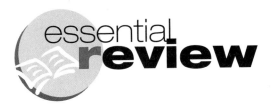

Complete the following review of Chapter 17, "Nail Structure and Growth," by circling the correct answer to each question.

1. The technical name for the nail is _____.

   a) onychauxis   b) onychia

   c) onyx   d) onychosis

2. A healthy nail appears slightly _____ in color.

   a) yellow   b) pink

   c) blue   d) purple

3. In an adult, the nail grows at an average of _____ inch per month.

   a) 1/8   b) 1/16

   c) 1/4   d) 3/8

4. The matrix bed is composed of matrix cells that produce the nail _____.

   a) lunula   b) plate

   c) grooves   d) mantle

5. The nail bed is supplied with many nerves and is attached to the nail plate by a thin layer of tissue called the _____.

   a) bed epithelium   b) hyponychium

   c) nail grooves   d) eponychium

6. The cuticle overlapping the lunula is the _____.

   a) mantle   b) hyponychium

   c) matrix   d) eponychium

7. Wavy rides or _____ are caused by uneven growth of the nails.

   a) furrows   b) depressions

   c) corrugations   d) pterygium

8. _____ on the nails are known as leukonychia.

   a) white spots   b) blue spots

   c) white stripes   d) vertical ridges

9. Atrophy or wasting away of the nails is also known as _____.

   a) onychauxis   b) onychatrophia

   c) onychophagy   d) pterygium

10. Bitten nails, a result of an acquired nervous habit, are known as _____.

   a) onychauxis   b) onychatrophia

   c) onychophagy   d) pterygium

essential review *continued*

11. A forward growth of the cuticle that adheres to the base of the nail is known as

_____.

a) onychauxis

b) onychatrophia

c) onychophagy

d) pterygium

12. Hangnails are treated by _____ .

a) hot oil manicures

b) filing straight across

c) avoiding polish use

d) firm use of metal pusher

13. Blue nails are usually a sign of _____.

a) a blood disorder

b) a lung disorder

c) poor blood circulation

d) a heart problem

14. A general term for a vegetable parasite is _____.

a) flagella

b) fungi

c) mold

d) fungus

15. Darkening of the fingernails or toenails is technically known as _____.

a) melanonychia

b) leukonychia

c) onychatrophia

d) onychauxis

16. Periodic shedding of one or more nails, in whole or in part, is known as _____.

a) paronychia

b) onychoptosis

c) onychatrophia

d) onychauxis

17. Onychocryptosis is the technical term for _____.

a) split nails

b) bitten nails

c) bruised nails

d) ingrown nails

18. An infectious and inflammatory condition of the tissues surrounding the nails is known as

_____.

a) onychia

b) onychomycosis

c) paronychia

d) onychocryptosis

19. The technical term for loosening of the nail without shedding or falling off is _____.

a) onycholysis

b) onychogryposis

c) onychomycosis

d) onychophosis

20. A growth of horny epithelium in the nail bed is known as _____.

a) onycholysis

b) onychogryposis

c) onychophyma

d) onychophosis

essential discoveries and accomplishments

In the space below, jot some notes about what concepts of this chapter were hardest for you to understand or remember. Imagine finding yourself suddenly in the role of "teacher" and consider what you would tell your "students" about these difficult concepts.

Share your *Essential Discoveries* with some of the other students in your class and ask if they are helpful to them. You may want to revise your notes based on good ideas shared by your peers. Under "Accomplishments," list at least three things you have accomplished since your last entry that relate to your career goals.

Discoveries:

_____

_____

_____

_____

_____

Accomplishments:

_____

_____

_____

_____

_____

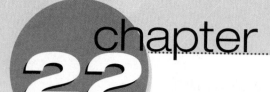

chapter

22

Manicuring and Pedicuring

essential **objectives**

After studying this chapter and completing the Essential Companion *components, you should be able to:*

1. List the abilities that make a good nail technician.

2. Identify the five basic nail shapes.

3. Demonstrate the proper use of implements, cosmetics, and materials used in manicuring and pedicuring.

4. Describe and demonstrate the different types of manicures.

5. Demonstrate massage techniques used when giving a manicure or pedicure.

6. Demonstrate the proper procedures and sanitary and safety precautions for a manicure and pedicure.

essential manicuring and pedicuring

Why are manicuring and pedicuring so important in my career as a cosmetologist?

It may help to understand a little of the history of manicuring in order to understand its relevance in today's society. The word *manicure* comes from the Latin word *manus* (which means "hand") and the word *cura* (which means "care"). So, manicuring means just that—to improve the appearance of the hands and nails. You need to be able to provide this important service to your clients, but you also must maintain your own hands and nails in the best possible condition. After all, you will be touching your clients with your hands during every service you offer. It is important that your nails are smooth and don't scratch a client's skin or scalp.

The early societies of Egypt and China considered long, polished, and colored fingernails as a mark of distinction between commoners and aristocrats. Nails were shaped with pumice stones and colored with vegetable dyes. In the late 1800s painted fingernails became a trend among the elite in Paris. Manicuring as a service and wearing nail polish became so popular in the 1920s that barber shops began to offer nail services to both men and women. By the late 1950s, most states began to require licensure for this special service.

essential concepts

What do I need to know about manicuring and pedicuring in order to provide a quality service?

As with other services you provide, you will need to thoroughly consult with each client to learn what his or her specific desires are for the nail service. You will need to be able to file and shape the nails to the desired shape. You must be able to gather and properly use all the implements and equipment required in the various nail procedures. You will learn the importance of being able to provide an effective hand and arm or foot massage in manicuring and pedicuring.

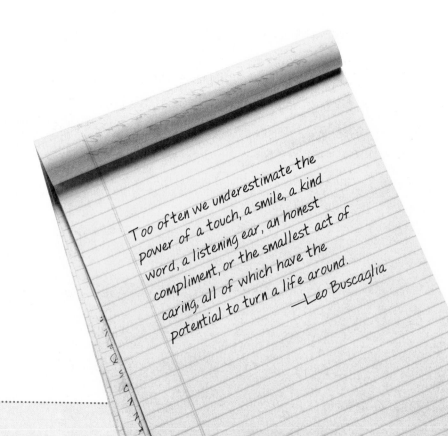

Too often we underestimate the power of a touch, a smile, a kind word, a listening ear, an honest compliment, or the smallest act of caring, all of which have the potential to turn a life around.

—Leo Buscaglia

essential experience

1

Windowpane—Nail Shapes

Windowpaning is the process of transferring key elements, points, or steps in a lesson into visual images that are hand sketched into the squares or "panes" of a matrix. Let your mind think in pictures and sketch the essential concepts printed in each of the following windowpanes. Don't be concerned with your artistic ability. Use lines and stick figures to depict the concepts requested.

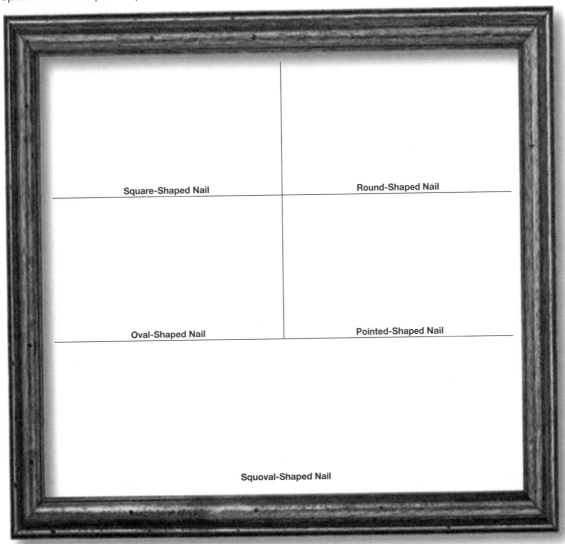

Square-Shaped Nail	Round-Shaped Nail
Oval-Shaped Nail	Pointed-Shaped Nail
Squoval-Shaped Nail	

essential
2 experience

Implements

Identify each of the manicuring implements depicted below.

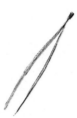

_____

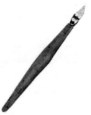

_____

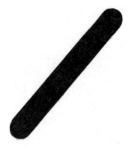

_____

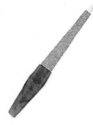

_____

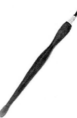

_____

_____

_____

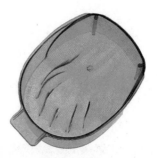

_____

essential
experience
3

Matching Exercise

Match the following essential terms with their identifying phrases or definition.

_____	Supply tray	**1.**	Liquid soap
_____	Paper cup	**2.**	Avoids infections of a minor cut
_____	Chamois	**3.**	Used to sanitize implements and the manicure table
_____	Cleanser	**4.**	Used to apply cosmetics to the nails
_____	Absorbent cotton	**5.**	Water temperature for a finger bath
_____	Disinfectant	**6.**	For repairing or covering broken, split, torn, or weak nails
_____	Mending tissue	**7.**	Removes creams from jars
_____	Antiseptic	**8.**	Used in finger bowls
_____	Spatula	**9.**	Found on a buffer
_____	Warm	**10.**	Used for holding cosmetics

essential
experience
4

Word Scramble

Scramble	Correct Word
alin life	_ _ _ _ _ _ _ _ _ _ *Clue:* Used for shaping and smoothing the free edge
litucce presinp	_ _ _ _ _ _ _ _ _ _ _ _ _ _ _ _ *Clue:* Used for trimming the cuticle
lian fubref	_ _ _ _ _ _ _ _ _ _ _ *Clue:* Used for buffing and polishing the nail
rengfi wblo	_ _ _ _ _ _ _ _ _ _ _ *Clue:* Holds warm, soapy water
tuclice hspure	_ _ _ _ _ _ _ _ _ _ _ _ _ _ _ *Clue:* Loosens and pushes back the cuticle
cirtleec retahe	_ _ _ _ _ _ _ _ _ _ _ _ _ _ _ *Clue:* Heats oil
ailn sbruh	_ _ _ _ _ _ _ _ _ _ *Clue:* Used for cleansing nails and fingertips
yeerm drbao	_ _ _ _ _ _ _ _ _ _ _ _ *Clue:* Used for shaping the free edge
yulpps ytar	_ _ _ _ _ _ _ _ _ _ _ _ *Clue:* Holds cosmetics for the nails
ezsewret	_ _ _ _ _ _ _ _ *Clue:* Used for lifting small bits of cuticle
rnienaotc	_ _ _ _ _ _ _ _ _ *Clue:* Holds clean absorbent cotton

essential experience
5

Crossword Puzzle

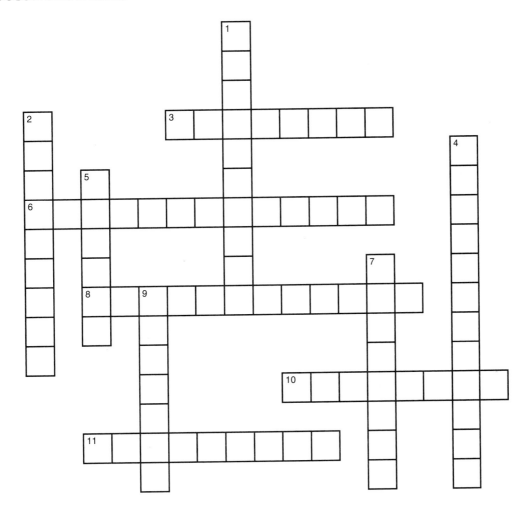

Across

3. Keeps tips looking white
6. Dissolves old polish
8. Corrects brittle nails and dry cuticles
10. Allows the nail polish to adhere more readily to the nail surface
11. Consist of detergent

Down

1. Lubricates the skin around the nail
2. In the form of a powder or paste
4. A styptic to stop bleeding of minor cuts
5. Contains hydrogen peroxide; removes stains
7. Designed to prevent nails from splitting or peeling
9. Contains acetone

essential
6 experience

Manicure Procedure

Put the following steps for a plain manicure in the appropriate order.

——————— Apply top or seal coat

——————— Apply base coat

——————— Apply instant nail dryer

——————— Apply polish

——————— Apply cuticle remover

——————— Apply cuticle oil or cream

——————— Bleach under free edge

——————— Choose color and mix polish

——————— Clean under free edge

——————— Cleanse nails

——————— Dry hands and nails thoroughly

——————— Dry fingertips

——————— Give hand and arm massage

——————— Immerse fingers of right hand

——————— Loosen cuticle

——————— Manicure right hand

——————— Perform post-service procedure

——————— Reexamine nails and cuticles

——————— Remove old polish

——————— Remove excess polish

——————— Repair split or broken nails

——————— Shape nails

——————— Soften cuticle

——————— Trim cuticle

essential
7 experience

Partners for Pedicure

Choose a partner and provide a pedicure service to each other. Rate each other's procedure according to the following evaluation form. Circle the numeric score you would assign the service you just received, using the following rating scale.

1 = Poor; 2 = Below Average; 3 = Average; 4 = Good; 5 = Excellent

1 2 3 4 5	**1.** You were seated comfortably and asked to remove shoes and socks or stockings.
1 2 3 4 5	**2.** All required equipment, implements, and materials were arranged.
1 2 3 4 5	**3.** Your feet were placed on a clean paper towel on footrest.
1 2 3 4 5	**4.** Nail technician's hands were washed and sanitized.
1 2 3 4 5	**5.** A basin was filled with warm water to cover ankles.
1 2 3 4 5	**6.** Antiseptic or liquid soap was added to the basin; both feet were placed in the bath for 3 to 5 minutes.
1 2 3 4 5	**7.** Feet were removed and wiped dry.
1 2 3 4 5	**8.** Old polish was thoroughly removed from the nails of both feet.
1 2 3 4 5	**9.** Toenails of left foot were clipped.
1 2 3 4 5	**10.** Toe separators were inserted.
1 2 3 4 5	**11.** Toenails were filed straight across, rounding them slightly at the corners to conform to the shape of the toes.
1 2 3 4 5	**12.** Foot file was used on ball and heel of left foot to remove dry skin and smooth down callus growths.
1 2 3 4 5	**13.** Toe separator was removed and left foot was placed in warm, soapy water.
1 2 3 4 5	**14.** Steps 9–13 were completed on the right foot.

1 2 3 4 5   **15.** Left foot was removed from basin, rinsed, dried, toe separators inserted.

1 2 3 4 5   **16.** Cuticle solvent was applied under free edge of each toenail of left foot with cotton-tipped orangewood stick.

1 2 3 4 5   **17.** Cuticle was gently loosened with the cotton-tipped orangewood stick. Cuticle was kept moist with additional lotion or water. Excessive pressure was not used. Cuticle was not cut.

1 2 3 4 5   **18.** Left foot was rinsed and dried.

1 2 3 4 5   **19.** Cream or lotions were applied.

1 2 3 4 5   **20.** Left foot was massaged and placed on a clean towel on floor.

1 2 3 4 5   **21.** Steps 15–20 were repeated on the right foot.

1 2 3 4 5   **22.** Lotion or cream was removed from toenails.

1 2 3 4 5   **23.** Base coat, two color coats, and top coat were applied.

1 2 3 4 5   **24.** Post-service steps were completed.

essential review

Using the following words, fill in the blanks below to form a thorough review of Chapter 22, "Manicuring and Pedicuring." Words or terms may be used more than once.

accidents	cut	metal	root
acetone	cuticle pusher	musk-scented	round
alkali	cuticles	nail brush	sanitation
analysis	electric	oil	sculptured
athlete's foot	finger bowl	open-toe	shinbone
biohazardous	fingertips	organic	solvent
waste	French	oval	squoval
bleaches	fringe	pedicuring	straight
circulatory	hand and arm	podiatrist	styptic
contagious	massage	pointed	trash container
contamination	hardeners	powdered alum	tweezers
corner	health	previous manicure	well-groomed
corners	humectants	protected	
cotton-tipped	jewelry	recommendations	
cura	manus	remove old polish	

1. The word manicure is derived from the Latin _____ which means hand and _____ which means care.

2. It is generally felt that the nails should be shaped to mirror the shape of the _____ .

3. A _____ is used for holding warm soapy water during a manicure.

4. An implement used for loosening and pushing back the cuticle is the _____ .

5. The implement used for cleansing the nails and fingertips with the aid of warm soapy water is a _____ .

6. _____ are used for lifting small bits of cuticle.

7. Never allow your hands to come in contact with the disinfectant solution used in manicuring, as this can cause _____ .

8. Cuticle removers are solutions of _____ , glycerin, and water used to soften and remove dead cuticle from around the nail.

9. Nail _____ are applied over nails, under the free edges, and on fingertips to remove stains.

essential
review *continued*

10. A _____ manicure polishes the free edge in an opaque color while the nail plate is polished or left a more translucent color.

11. Nail polish thinner contains _____ .

12. Nail _____ are designed to prevent nails from splitting or peeling.

13. During a manicure, if a client is accidentally cut, apply a _____ .

14. Hand creams are made up of emollients and _____ .

15. In some states or provinces it is a violation of sanitary codes to have _____ implements on your table when not in use.

16. When giving a professional manicure, all rules of _____ must be followed.

17. Do not ask the client to sit at the table with the remains of the _____ in sight.

18. The first step in the manicure procedure is to _____ .

19. File nails with a file or emery board, filing from _____ to center.

20. Use a _____ orangewood stick, dipped in soapy water, to clean under the free edge.

21. When using a cuticle pusher, use light pressure so the tissue at the _____ of the nail will not be injured.

22. If the cuticle is trimmed closer than necessary, a _____ of loose skin may be left around the nail after the manicure.

23. Observing safety rules in manicuring can be of great help in preventing _____ and injury to the client or nail technician.

24. Nails shapes can be divided into five types: oval, pointed, square, squoval, or _____ .

25. The ideal nail shape is the _____ nail.

26. The _____ nail is well suited for thin, delicate hands.

27. Formaldehyde _____ use keratin fibers to strengthen the nail.

28. A hand massage with each manicure will keep the hands flexible, _____ , and smooth.

29. A special service that may be added to the plain manicure is the _____ .

30. A manicure given with a portable device operated by a small motor is an _____ manicure.

31. Brittle nails and dry cuticles are treated with an _____ manicure.

32. During a men's manicure, file the nails either _____ or square.

essential review *continued*

33. Before applying polish, ask the client to replace _____, locate car keys, pay for the service and any applicable retail products, and put on any outer clothing such as sweaters or jackets.

34. Aluminum salt is used as a _____ to stop bleeding when accidental cuts occur during a manicure.

35. Polish remover containing _____ will damage plastic artificial nails.

36. The care of the feet, toes, and toenails is called _____ .

37. Abnormal foot conditions, such as corns, calluses, and ingrown nails, are best treated by a qualified _____ .

38. When making a pedicure appointment, suggest that the client wear _____ shoes or sandals so that the polish will not smear at the completion of the service.

39. A manicure or pedicure should not be administered to a person with a _____ disease or skin condition.

40. File toenails with an emery board _____ across, rounding them slightly at the corners.

41. To avoid ingrown toenails, avoid filing into the _____ of the nails.

42. During a pedicure, do not _____ the cuticle.

43. During a foot massage, when massaging from the ankle to the knee, do not massage over the _____ and above the knee.

44. Your _____ should have a lid that can be operated by a foot pedal.

45. During a nail service consultation, you will discuss the client's general _____, the health of his or her nails and skin, the client's lifestyle and needs, and the nail services you can offer.

46. A nail service consultation consists of two parts: _____ and _____ .

47. Clients with arthritis should have their hands held gently during the service, while clients who have a _____ disease, such as varicose veins, should be massaged very carefully.

48. A square nail with the ends (or corners) slightly rounded or taken off is known as _____ .

49. A citrus or _____ hand cream is recommended over a flowery one for a man's hand massage.

50. Any blood-contaminated disposable implements and materials should be placed in a sealed plastic bag marked _____ .

essential
discoveries and accomplishments

In the space below, jot some notes about what concepts of this chapter were hardest for you to understand or remember. Imagine finding yourself suddenly in the role of "teacher" and consider what you would tell your "students" about these difficult concepts.

Share your *Essential Discoveries* with some of the other students in your class and ask if they are helpful to them. You may want to revise your notes based on good ideas shared by your peers. Under "Accomplishments," list at least three things you have accomplished since your last entry that relate to your career goals.

Discoveries:

_____

_____

_____

_____

_____

Accomplishments:

_____

_____

_____

_____

_____

Advanced Nail Techniques

After studying this chapter and completing the Essential Companion *components, you should be able to:*

1. List the pre-service and post-service steps of an artificial nail procedure.

2. Describe the various types of artificial nails: a) tips, b) wraps, c) acrylic nails, and d) gels.

3. Explain the chemistry of acrylic nails.

4. Demonstrate the basic procedures for applying: a) tips, b) wraps, c) acrylic nails, and d) gels.

5. List the safety precautions that must be followed when applying artificial nails.

essential advanced nail techniques

Why do I need to learn about advanced nail techniques to be successful?

The nail industry experienced great expansion when the first acrylic artificial nail extensions were introduced in the early 1970s. The popular singer and actress Cher started a trend of very long nails which were squared off at the ends. By the 1980s, manufacturers had developed products with which to create natural-looking artificial nails. It was then that the nail industry became the fastest growing area in the entire field of cosmetology, and it's still growing today. Cosmetologists who fine-tune their skills in manicuring, pedicuring, and advanced nail techniques can earn a very good income.

essential concepts of advanced nail techniques

What do I need to know about advanced nail techniques in order to provide a quality service?

There are no evil thoughts except one: the refusal to think.
—Ayn Rand

You will need to become familiar and experienced with a variety of advanced nail techniques from nail tips and wraps to acrylic nail applications. It has been said that with today's technology, there is no reason for anyone who wants long beautiful nails not to have them. As a professional cosmetologist, you must prepare to deliver just those services that will meet that need.

essential
1 experience

Windowpane

Windowpaning is the process of transferring key elements, points, or steps in a lesson into visual images that are hand sketched into the squares or "panes" of a matrix. Let your mind think in pictures and sketch the essential concepts printed in each of the following windowpanes. Don't be concerned with your artistic ability. Use lines and stick figures to depict the concepts requested.

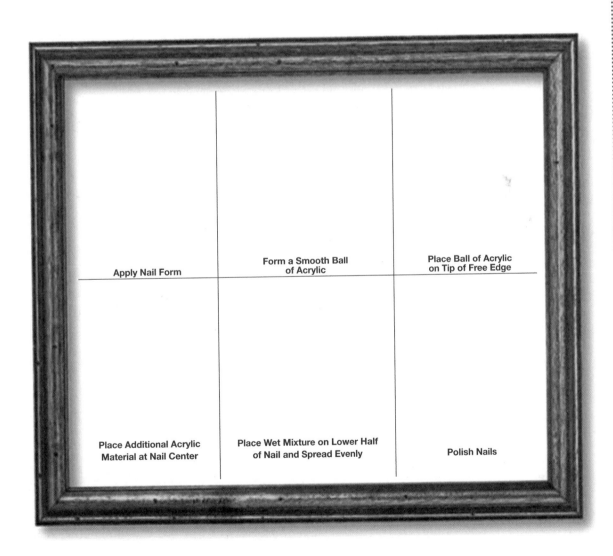

Apply Nail Form	Form a Smooth Ball of Acrylic	Place Ball of Acrylic on Tip of Free Edge
Place Additional Acrylic Material at Nail Center	Place Wet Mixture on Lower Half of Nail and Spread Evenly	Polish Nails

essential
experience
2

Pre- and Post-Service Procedures

Number the following steps for an advanced nail technique pre- and post-service procedure.

Pre-Service Procedure

_____ Greet your client and ask her to wash her hands with soap and warm water. Wash your hands as well, using a waterless hand sanitizer gel or wipe. Dry hands and nails thoroughly with a clean and/or disposable towel.

_____ Completely immerse all implements in an EPA-registered, hospital-level disinfectant for the required time (usually 20 minutes). Use tongs or rubber gloves to avoid skin contact with the disinfectant.

_____ Disinfect all working surfaces. Spray with an EPA-registered disinfectant that is approved by your state or province. Allow surfaces to remain wet for 10 minutes and then wipe dry. Spray again and allow the surfaces to air dry.

_____ Perform a client consultation. Fill out a client card. If you determine that it is safe to proceed with the service, discuss your client's needs and wants.

_____ Rinse the implements in plain warm water, taking care to wash away all traces of soap. Dry thoroughly with a clean and/or disposable towel.

_____ Wash your hands with liquid soap and warm water. Rinse well and dry with a clean and/or disposable towel.

_____ Refill all disposable materials—abrasive (file), orangewood stick, cotton balls, and other such materials—on the manicuring table. These materials are discarded after they have been used.

_____ Sanitize the manicure table by wiping with disinfectant or sanitizing solution.

_____ Rinse all implements with cool running water, then wash with soap and warm water.

essential
experience *continued*
2

_____ Wrap the manicuring cushion with a clean and/or disposable towel.

_____ Remove the implements from the disinfectant solution with tongs or while wearing rubber gloves and rinse them well in water. Wipe them dry with a clean and/or disposable towel to prevent rusting.

_____ Set up the standard manicuring table, adding the items you need for the advanced nail service you are performing.

_____ Follow your state or province regulations for storing sanitized manicuring implements (usually sealed containers or closed cabinet sanitizer).

Post-Service Procedure

_____ Clean the table and surrounding area. Allow enough time to restore the basic setup.

_____ Book another appointment with the client.

_____ Sanitize the table and disinfect implements. Perform the complete pre-service sanitation procedure.

_____ Offer retail products to the client.

_____ Discard all used materials in a closed pail.

essential
experience
3

Nail Tip Procedure

Nail Tip Procedure

_____ Select the proper size tip. Make sure it completely covers the nail plate from sidewall to sidewall but never covers more than half the length of the nail. Trim the tip to the right size if the well covers too much of the nail.

_____ Proceed with any other service that may be desired. Tips are seldom worn without an additional service such as wraps, acrylics, or gels. If your client is only wearing tips as a temporary service, add a drop of cuticle oil to each nail and then buff.

_____ Trim the nail to the desired length, using a tip clipper or large nail clippers. Cut from one side, then the other, if you are using the nail clippers. Cutting the tip straight across weakens the plastic.

_____ Apply nail antiseptic to remove the remaining natural oil and to dehydrate the nail for better adhesion. Again, begin with the little finger. (If you accidentally touch the nails after you apply antiseptic, you must clean them again and reapply antiseptic.)

_____ Remove any old polish from the client's nails, working from the little finger to thumb.

_____ Apply adhesive on the nail plate to cover the area where the tip will be placed. Do not let adhesive run onto the skin. Apply adhesive from the middle of the nail plate to the free edge. An alternate method is to apply adhesive to the well of the tip. This may ensure that fewer air bubbles are trapped in the adhesive.

_____ Slide on the tip. Use a stop, rock, and hold procedure:
Stop: Find the stop against the free edge at a 45-degree angle.
Rock: Rock the tip on slowly.
Hold: Hold in place for 5 to 10 seconds until dry.

essential
experience *continued*

_____ Shape the nail.

_____ Apply a bead of adhesive to the seam between the natural nail plate and the tip to strengthen the stress point.

_____ Buff the tip for a perfect blend between the natural nail plate and the tip extension. There should be no visible line or cloudiness between the two.

_____ Buff the nails to remove shine and any natural oils. Remove the dust.

_____ Blend the tip into the natural nail. File the shine off the tip, keeping the file flat on the nail at all times. Never hold the file at an angle, because doing so can form a groove in the nail plate.

_____ Push back the cuticle.

_____ Perform the post-service procedure.

essential
4experience

Word Scramble

Scramble	Correct Word
aosylrev	_ _ _ _ _ _ _ _ _ *Clue:* Any wraps, acrylic, or gel applied over the entire natural nail plate or tip
erirmp	_ _ _ _ _ _ _ *Clue:* Substance that improves adhesion, or attachment, and prepares the nail surface for bonding with the acrylic material
ernmoom	_ _ _ _ _ _ _ _ *Clue:* Substance made up of many small molecules that are not attached to one another
irnguc	_ _ _ _ _ _ _ *Clue:* Hardening process that occurs when powdered and liquid acrylic are combined to form nails
istp	_ _ _ _ _ *Clue:* Pre-formed artificial nails applied to the tips of the natural nails
mryeolp	_ _ _ _ _ _ _ _ *Clue:* Hard substance formed by combining many small molecules, usually in a long chain-like structure
nacricnlabe	_ _ _ _ _ _ _ _ _ _ _ *Clue:* Redefining the shape of the acrylic nail during a fill procedure
sciracly	_ _ _ _ _ _ _ _ *Clue:* Sculptured nails; artificial nails created by combining a liquid acrylic product with a powdered product to form a soft ball that can easily be molded into a nail shape

essential
experience *continued*
4

Word Scramble (continued)

Scramble	Correct Word
slge	_ _ _ _ *Clue:* Strong, durable artificial nails that are brushed on the nail plate
spwar	_ _ _ _ _ *Clue:* Corrective treatments that form a protective coating for damaged or fragile nails
ytaasltc	_ _ _ _ _ _ _ _ *Clue:* Any substance having the power to increase the velocity of a chemical reaction

essential experience
5

Word Search

After determining the correct words from the clues provided, locate the words in the word search puzzle.

Word	Clue
_____	Sculptured nails
_____	Acrylic nails applied directly to the natural nail surface or nail tip
_____	Hardening process for acrylic nails
_____	Created by dipping fingernails into acrylic powder
_____	Acrylic product applied to a new growth of fingernail
_____	Gel nail that hardens when exposed to a special light source, either ultraviolet or halogen
_____	Substance made from many small molecules that are not attached to each other
_____	Corrective treatment that forms a protective coating for damaged or fragile nails
_____	Gel nail that hardens when an activator or accelerator is sprayed or brushed on
_____	Any wrap, acrylic, or gel applied over the entire natural nail plate
_____	Hard substance formed by combining many small molecules, usually in a long chain-like structure
_____	Point where the nail plate meets the tip before it is glued to the nail
_____	Substance that improves adhesion and prepares the surface for bonding
_____	Redefining the shape of acrylic nails during a fill procedure

```
A  C  R  Y  L  I  C  O  V  E  R  L  A  Y  S
C  M  Q  R  E  M  Y  L  O  P  R  O  E  M  L
R  D  C  H  G  N  I  R  U  C  E  W  G  C  I
Y  Y  O  F  D  X  N  Z  W  P  B  Y  M  J  A
L  M  T  R  E  M  I  R  P  F  A  Q  F  S  N
I  M  P  G  R  L  B  Q  W  Z  L  A  Z  F  D
C  O  J  P  U  E  H  F  K  N  A  C  V  G  E
N  N  V  X  C  Z  V  S  N  D  N  N  Z  U  P
A  O  Q  U  -  W  D  U  W  T  C  Z  E  S  P
I  M  P  O  T  S  N  O  I  T  I  S  O  P  I
L  E  G  T  H  G  I  L  -  O  N  L  J  Q  D
S  R  F  A  G  M  K  H  N  S  G  L  R  E  C
G  R  G  N  I  P  P  A  R  W  L  I  A  N  P
Y  W  I  S  L  N  H  S  W  J  Q  F  T  W  R
```

essential experience

6

Client Consultation

Develop several open-ended questions that you would use in a client consultation prior to an advanced nail technique service and write them in the space provided.

1. _____

2. _____

3. _____
_____

4. _____

5. _____

6. _____
_____
_____

7. _____
_____
_____

8. _____

9. _____
_____

essential
experience
7

Acrylic Nail Procedure

In your own words list the steps for applying acrylic nails in the space provided.

Procedure

1. _____

2. _____

3. _____
   _____

4. _____
   _____

5. _____

6. _____
   _____
   _____
   _____
   _____

7. _____
   _____
   _____
   _____

8. _____
   _____

9. _____
   _____
   _____
   _____

essential
experience
7
continued

10. _____
_____

11. _____
_____
_____
_____
_____

12. _____
_____
_____
_____

13. _____
_____
_____
_____

14. _____

15. _____
_____

16. _____
_____

17. _____

18. _____

19. _____
_____
_____

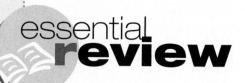

essential
review

Using the following words, fill in the blanks below to form a thorough review of Chapter 23, "Advanced Nail Techniques." Words or terms may be used more than once or not at all.

5 to 10	cloudy	mesh	rebalancing
10 to 20	curing	metal pusher	rebuffing
abrasive	cyanoacrylate	monomer	remove old polish
acetone	environment	nail art	rotating
acid	extend	nail biting	slick
antiseptic	fibers	nail plate	soaked
atomized spray	flush	observations	solvent
badly shaped	four	overlays	splitting
buffed	free edge	position stop	temporary
catalyst	grooved	post-service	tongs
chain-like	hospital-level	powdered	transparent
chemical	lifting	pre-beveled	underside
consistency	linear	pre-formed	

1. One advantage of artificial nails is to improve the appearance of very short or _____ nails.

2. The first step in a pre-service procedure includes brushing all _____ items and any open hinges of implements.

3. When sanitizing advanced nail service implements, they should be completely immersed in an EPA-registered, _____ disinfectant for the required time.

4. _____ or rubber gloves are used to avoid skin contact with disinfectant.

5. In preparing your manicure table for an advanced nail service, be sure to refill all disposable material such as the _____ (file), orangewood stick, cotton balls, and other such materials.

6. When performing the client consultation, be sure to record your _____ and the client's responses on a client record card.

7. An important part of the _____ procedure is booking another appointment with your client to ensure proper maintenance of her new nails.

8. One of the most popular advanced nail techniques is nail tips, which are _____ artificial nails applied to the tips of the natural fingernails.

essential review *continued*

9. Usually tips are combined with another artificial nail service such as wraps, acrylic, or gel _____ .

10. All nail tips have a well that serves as the point of contact with the _____ .

11. The _____ is the point where the nail plate meets the tip before it is glued to the nail.

12. Tips that are _____ require less filing on the natural nail after application.

13. The first step in any nail service procedure is to _____ from the client's nails, working from the little finger to the thumb.

14. In the stop, rock, and hold procedure, the stop step means finding the stop against the _____ at a 45-degree angle.

15. In the stop, rock, and hold procedure, the hold step means to hold the tip in place for _____ seconds until dry.

16. Clients wearing nail tips will need weekly or biweekly manicures to allow for regluing and _____ .

17. When removing nail tips after soaking, use a fresh orangewood stick or a _____ to slide off the softened tips.

18. Silk nail wraps give a smooth, even appearance to the nail and become almost _____ when the adhesive is applied.

19. Fiberglass is a very thin synthetic _____ with a loose weave that makes it easy for adhesive to penetrate.

20. Paper wraps are made of very thin paper and dissolve in both acetone and non-acetone remover, so they are considered a _____ service.

21. In performing a nail wrap procedure, the nail should be sprayed or wiped with a nail _____ to remove the remaining natural oil and to dehydrate the nail for better adhesion.

22. In applying nail wraps, it is important to apply a protective base coat to the top and _____ of the free edge of the nail and allow it to dry completely before applying nail enamel.

23. Fabric wraps require glue fills after two weeks and glue and fabric fills will be necessary after _____ weeks.

24. Liquid nail wrap is a polish made with tiny _____ designed to strengthen and preserve the nail as it grows.

25. Acrylic nails are artificial nails that are created by combining a liquid acrylic product with a _____ product.

essential review *continued*

26. Acrylics can be used to strengthen or _____ the nail or to repair weak, bitten, or torn nails.

27. A _____ is a substance made up of many small molecules that are not attached to one another.

28. A polymer is a hard substance formed by combining many small molecules, usually in a long _____ structure.

29. A _____ is any substance having the power to increase the velocity (speed) of a chemical reaction.

30. When the catalyst "explodes" as it comes in contact with the monomer, it causes heat which creates a hardening process called _____ .

31. Acrylics can be created using one-color powder for the entire nail or by using pink powder on the nail plate and white powder for the _____ to produce a French manicure look.

32. _____ primer is widely used to help bind the acrylic to the natural nail.

33. Overly primed nails can become too _____ and can cause the acrylic to lift.

34. When applying acrylic nails, dip the brush into the liquid mixture, wipe any excess material on the side of the bowl, and immediately dip the tip of the brush into the powder, _____ it slightly as it is drawn toward you to form a smooth ball of acrylic.

35. During the course of a fill, the shape of the nail should be defined with a process called _____ .

36. If an acrylic nail is badly chipped or cracked, your choice is to file a V shape into the crack or to file _____ to remove the crack if there is enough length on the extension.

37. To remove an acrylic nail, begin by soaking the nail in a _____ specified by the manufacturer or your instructor.

38. Gels have a _____ very similar to that of acrylic nails, but they require a separate catalyst to ensure hardening.

39. No-light gels harden when an activator or accelerator is sprayed or brushed on, or when they are _____ in water.

40. UV gels must be _____ off layer by layer and will not soak off in acetone.

41. No-light gels can be soaked off with _____ .

42. Most dipped nails do not rely on an acrylic monomer but use instead a _____ which is a fast-setting glue which comes in different viscosities and can be applied in several ways.

essential review *continued*

43. Advanced technology allows for exciting custom designs, which has made _____ one of the most popular add-on services salons can offer.

44. Do not use a nipper to clip away loose acrylic as it may make the _____ problem worse and can damage the nail plate.

45. Check the primer for clarity on a regular basis to make sure it is not contaminated with bacteria, which will be evident if the primer is _____ in appearance.

46. Tacky-backed striping tape helps you create more _____ or graphic designs when applying nail art.

47. An airbrush and compressor combine air and paint to form an _____ for painting on nails.

48. Artificial nail applications can be helpful in overcoming the habit of _____ .

49. Artificial nails can protect nails against _____ or breakage.

50. One national skill standard applies to artificial nail techniques in conducting services in a safe _____ and taking measures to prevent the spread of infectious and contagious disease.

essential
discoveries and
accomplishments

In the space below, jot some notes about what concepts of this chapter were hardest for you to understand or remember. Imagine finding yourself suddenly in the role of "teacher" and consider what you would tell your "students" about these difficult concepts.

Share your *Essential Discoveries* with some of the other students in your class and ask if they are helpful to them. You may want to revise your notes based on good ideas shared by your peers. Under "Accomplishments," list at least three things you have accomplished since your last entry that relate to your career goals.

Discoveries:

_____

_____

_____

_____

_____

Accomplishments:

_____

_____

_____

_____

_____

The Salon Business

essential **objectives**

After studying this chapter and completing the Essential Companion *components, you should be able to:*

1. Describe the two ways in which you may go into business for yourself.

2. List the factors to consider when opening a salon.

3. Name and describe the types of ownership under which a salon may operate.

4. Explain the importance of keeping accurate business records.

5. Discuss the importance of the reception area to a salon's success.

6. Demonstrate good salon telephone techniques.

7. List the most effective forms of salon advertising.

essential
salon
business

Is business knowledge really so important to someone who just wants to be a hair designer?

Absolutely! Even if you never own your own salon, you need to understand the key principles of building and operating a business to ensure your own success. However, most individuals who enter this exciting field dream of owning their own salon one day. The fact is that more than a few graduates actually turn that dream into reality. The more you know about managing and operating a sufficient business, the more valuable you become to your future employers.

essential
concepts

What do I need to know about the salon business in order to be successful?

There are many factors to consider before taking the step into ownership or even management. A knowledge of business principles, bookkeeping, business laws, insurance, salesmanship, and psychology is crucial for the successful salon owner or manager. Serving people is one thing; managing people is quite another. Just knowing about business is not enough. You need to develop leadership, self-control, and sensitivity. This whole area of business calls for planning, supervision, control, evaluation, and above all teamwork.

When you make a mistake, don't look back at it long. Take the reason of the thing into your mind, and then look forward. Mistakes are lessons of wisdom. The past cannot be changed. The future is yet in your power.
—Mary Pickford

essential
1 experience

Salon Research

Research at least five salons in the area where you may want to work. Your mission is to determine which salon is most suited to your needs. Rate each category on a scale of 1 to 10, with 10 being considered the best. Explain your rating. Use the chart below to track your findings.

Category	Salon 1	Salon 2	Salon 3	Salon 4	Salon 5
Location/Active Business Nearby					
Demographics/ Income Area					
Adequate Parking					
Direct Competition Nearby					
Exterior Appearance and Design (attractive)					
Interior Appearance and Design (attractive and efficient)					
Retail Sales Awareness					

essential
2 experience

Matching

Match each of the following essential terms with its definition.

_____ Local regulations

_____ Federal law

_____ State law

_____ Income tax law

_____ Insurance

1. Covers sales taxes, licenses, and employee compensation.

2. Covered by both state and federal government.

3. Covers building renovations.

4. Covers malpractice, premises liability, fire, burglary and theft, and business interruption.

5. Covers Social Security, unemployment compensation, cosmetics and luxury tax, and OSHA.

essential
3 experience

Income and Expense

Assume the following facts:

- Your monthly revenue goal is $10,000.
- The ticket average in your salon is $20.00 per client.
- Your salon is open 5 days per week or an average of 22 days per month.

Based on this information, determine how many clients you will have to serve per day and how many stylists you will have to employ to reach your revenue goal.

_____

_____

_____

Once you have obtained the above information, apply the percentages taken from the budget of your text to the $10,000 gross revenue to determine what your salon profit will be for the month.

Salaries	$10,000 × 53.5%	=	$_____
Rent	$10,000 × 13%	=	$_____
Supplies	$10,000 × 5%	=	$_____
Advertising	$10,000 × 3%	=	$_____
Depreciation	$10,000 × 3%	=	$_____
Laundry	$10,000 × 1%	=	$_____
Cleaning	$10,000 × 1%	=	$_____
Utilities	$10,000 × 1%	=	$_____
Repairs	$10,000 × 1.5%	=	$_____
Insurance	$10,000 × .75%	=	$_____
Telephone	$10,000 × .75%	=	$_____
Miscellaneous	$10,000 × 1.5%	=	$_____
	Total Expenses		$_____
	Net Profit		$_____

Now, consider what would happen if you were unable to stay within the recommended guidelines of your budget. Perhaps your rent is more than the amount above. Maybe you are having to pay more for a cleaning crew or you have several telephone lines and your telephone bill runs around $300 per month. It is important to consider all these factors when setting up a business because the only way to make more money is to increase revenue, or reduce expenses, or a combination of both.

essential
4 experience

Daily Revenue Report Form

On a separate sheet of paper, design a form on which you would track your clients on a daily basis. The form would record their services, retail sales, total sales, and possibly other items as well. You might want to track how the client heard about your salon or other data that would help you analyze your business.

essential
5 experience

Job Descriptions

On a separate sheet(s) of paper, write a position description for a stylist and a receptionist in your salon. Be thorough and specific. Outline their general responsibilities as well as their specific duties.

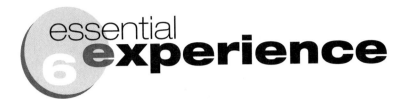

Advertising

In the space provided, design a 3" × 5" newspaper ad for your salon.

In the space provided, write a 30-second radio ad promoting your salon and its services.

_____

_____

_____

_____

_____

_____

_____

essential 7 experience

Crossword Puzzle

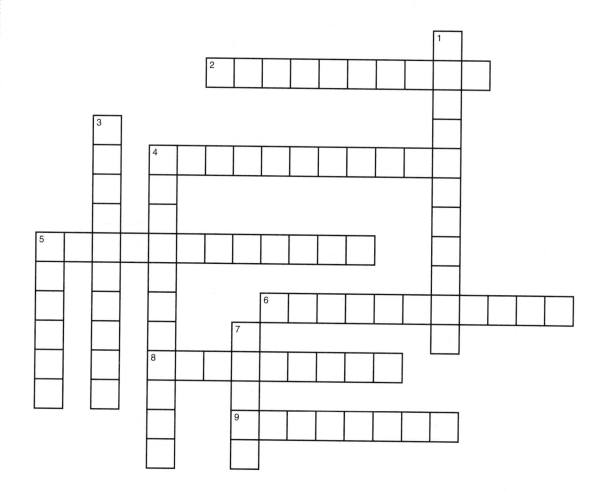

Across

2. Proprietor is owner and manager
4. Supplies used in the daily business operations
5. The quarterback of the salon
6. Should be 3 percent of your gross income
8. Complaints are often handled on this
9. Largest expense in the salon

Down

1. Ownership is shared by two or more people
3. Advertising that allows for close contact with the potential client
4. Ownership is shared by stockholders
5. Supplies sold to the client
7. Must contain all provisions that pertain to the landlord and tenant

essential
8 experience

Interviewing Personnel

Select a partner and role-play interviewing that person for employment in your salon.
Prepare in advance a list of questions you wish to ask him or her. List the questions and
his or her responses below.

_____

_____

_____

_____

_____

_____

_____

_____

_____

_____

_____

_____

_____

_____

_____

_____

_____

_____

_____

_____

essential review

Complete the following review of Chapter 24, "The Salon Business," by circling the correct answer to each question.

1. In order to obtain financing when opening a salon, it is necessary to have a/an

_____ .

   a) cosmetology license   b) credit card

   c) business plan   d) instructor's license

2. A charter from the state is required if the ownership is a/an _____ .

   a) partnership   b) corporation

   c) individual   d) co-owner

3. _____ advertising allows for closer contact with the potential clients.

   a) direct mail   b) television

   c) classified ads   d) radio

4. Social Security, unemployment compensation or insurance, and cosmetics and luxury tax

payments are covered by _____ .

   a) federal law   b) insurance

   c) state law   d) local regulations

5. Salon owners should have a general knowledge of _____ .

   a) equipment repair   b) fashion trends

   c) business principles   d) plumbing

6. Salon owners purchase insurance policies to protect themselves against lawsuits for

_____ .

   a) loss of clients   b) increases in rent

   c) loss of employees   d) malpractice

7. When the proprietor is owner and manager, the ownership is a/an _____ .

   a) partnership   b) corporation

   c) individual   d) co-owner

8. The largest expense in operating a salon is _____ .

   a) salaries   b) rent

   c) advertising   d) supplies

9. Supplies that are sold to the client are known as _____ supplies .

   a) consumption   b) cleaning

   c) retail   d) office

essential review *continued*

10. When selecting a location for a salon, consider _____ .

   a) services to be offered   b) demographics

   c) salon policies   d) staff to be hired

11. Supplies used in daily business operations are known as _____ supplies.

   a) consumption   b) cleaning

   c) retail   d) office

12. The layout of the salon should be planned for maximum _____ .

   a) efficiency   b) aisle space

   c) beauty   d) storage space

13. The "quarterback" of the salon is the _____ .

   a) manager   b) stylist

   c) receptionist   d) nail tech

14. The flow of operational services in the salon should be directed to the _____ area.

   a) shampoo   b) nail tech

   c) styling   d) reception

15. When booking appointments, services are sold in terms of _____ .

   a) time   b) client preferences

   c) salon size   d) stylist preferences

16. When listening to a client's complaint, avoid _____ .

   a) being sympathetic   b) apologizing

   c) promising refunds   d) interrupting

17. Three percent of a salon's gross income should be spent on _____ .

   a) salaries   b) rent

   c) advertising   d) supplies

18. A dramatic, but expensive medium of advertising is _____ .

   a) direct mail   b) television

   c) classified ads   d) radio

19. An important part of the salon business is handled over the _____ .

   a) Internet   b) telephone

   c) radio   d) intercom

20. Building renovations are usually covered by _____ .

   a) federal law   b) insurance

   c) state law   d) local regulations

essential discoveries and accomplishments

In the space below, jot some notes about what concepts of this chapter were hardest for you to understand or remember. Imagine finding yourself suddenly in the role of "teacher" and consider what you would tell your "students" about these difficult concepts.

Share your *Essential Discoveries* with some of the other students in your class and ask if they are helpful to them. You may want to revise your notes based on good ideas shared by your peers. Under "Accomplishments," list at least three things you have accomplished since your last entry that relate to your career goals.

Discoveries:

_____

_____

_____

_____

_____

Accomplishments:

_____

_____

_____

_____

_____

_____

Seeking Employment

essential objectives

After studying this chapter and completing the Essential Companion *components, you should be able to:*

1. Discuss the essentials of becoming test-wise.

2. Explain the steps involved in preparing for employment.

3. List and describe the different types of salon businesses.

4. Write an achievement-oriented resume and prepare an employment portfolio.

5. Explain how to explore the job market and research potential employers.

6. Be prepared to complete an effective employment interview.

essential
employment
seeking

Why do I need to learn about seeking employment while I am still in training?

Planning your career is an essential part of planning your life. If you set a goal on the first day of school to become a successful salon owner or a well-known, international platform artist, you must begin your journey toward that goal by obtaining your first career-related position. It is important for you to recognize that when you complete your course of study, your training has really just begun. You have become a student in life-long learning. Therefore, that first job needs to be suited for your interests, your talents, and your goals. In addition, it should provide opportunities for your continued growth and professional development. It is not realistic to believe you can obtain your license and find exactly what you are looking for on your first job inquiry. By beginning your search while you are in school, it is far more likely that you will secure an appropriate position upon graduation.

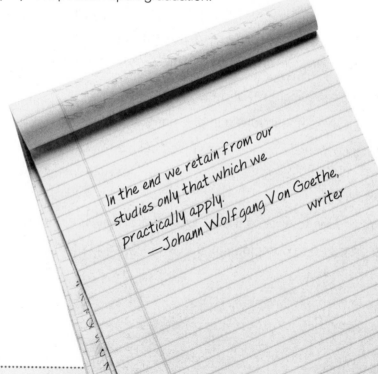

In the end we retain from our studies only that which we practically apply.
—Johann Wolfgang Von Goethe, writer

essential concepts of seeking employment

What do I need to know about seeking employment in order to achieve success in my career?

In addition to developing important personal characteristics such as a positive attitude, desire, and commitment, you will need to identify your talents, skills, and interests to determine the type of salon for which you are best suited. You will learn how to target those salons and observe them in action to confirm whether you want to pursue an employment interview. You must learn to develop an action-oriented resume that will catch the potential employer's eye in a few short seconds. You will need to properly prepare for the ever-important job interview. In our society, first impressions matter a great deal. You may have already learned in life that the best qualified applicant does not always get the best job. In fact, the job often goes to the applicant who projects the best image and comes across best during the interview. Thus, learning how to prepare for the interview and how to present yourself during the interview are critical to obtaining the most appropriate position upon graduation.

essential
1 experience

Personal Data Page

In preparation for accurate and prompt completion of an employment application, it is beneficial to prepare a personal data page that contains the same general information. Gather all the necessary information ahead of time and list it on the form below. It will then be easy to transfer the applicable information to the application form used by your potential employer.

Name: _____ Over Age 18: _____ Yes _____ No

Address: _____

Telephone: _____ E-mail: _____

Position Desired: _____ Date Available: _____

Education

High School Attended: _____ Graduated: ____Yes ____ No

Post-secondary: _____ Diploma: ____Yes ____No

Post-secondary: _____ Diploma: ____Yes ____No

Post-secondary: _____ Diploma: ____Yes ____No

Employment History

Where: _____ When: _____

Position: _____ Reason Left: _____

Where: _____ When: _____

Position: _____ Reason Left: _____

Where: _____ When: _____

Position: _____ Reason Left: _____

Significant Skills: _____

Awards and Recognitions: _____

essential
experience
2

Mind Map—The Steps in Seeking Employment

Mind mapping creates a free-flowing outline of material or information. Using the central or key point of seeking employment, diagram the different procedural steps you will need to complete in order to obtain the best possible position. Use terms, pictures, and symbols as desired. Using color will increase your retention of the material. Keep your mind open. Don't worry about where a line or word should go as the organization of the map will usually take care of itself.

essential
3 experience

Windowpane—Clinic Achievements

Windowpaning is the process of transferring key elements, points, or steps in a lesson into visual images that are hand sketched into the squares or "panes" of a matrix. Let your mind think in pictures and sketch the essential concepts printed in each of the following windowpanes. Don't be concerned with your artistic ability. Use lines and stick figures to depict the concepts requested for creating an achievement-oriented resume.

Total Regular Clients	Clients Served Weekly	% Clinic in Texture Services
Client Ticket Average	Client Retention Rate	% Clinic in Retail
% Clinic in Haircolor	Attendance Record	Other Accomplishments

essential
4 experience

Cover Letter

Using the format described in your chapter, write a cover letter to accompany your resume when applying for a job.

Date _____

Your Name _____

Your Address _____

City/State _____

Salon Name _____

Salon Address _____

City/State _____

Dear _____

_____

_____

_____

_____

_____

_____

_____

_____

Very cordially yours,

(Signature here)

Your Name

Enclosure

essential
experience
5

Interview Preparation

Listed below are several potential questions that may be asked during your interview. Using the space provided, answer the questions to the best of your ability. This exercise will help you be more thoroughly prepared for that important interview.

What did you like best about your training? _____

_____

Are you punctual and regular in attendance? _____

What skills do you feel are your strongest? _____

_____

What skills do you feel are your weakest? _____

_____

Are you a team player? _____ Please explain: _____

_____

Are you flexible? _____ Please explain: _____

_____

What are your career goals? _____

_____

What days/hours are you available to work? _____

Do you have your own transportation? _____

What obstacles, if any, would prevent you from keeping your commitment to full-time employment? _____

_____

What assets will you bring to the salon and this position? _____

_____

Who is the most important person you have met in your work/education experience and why?

_____

Explain some strategies you would use in handling a difficult client. _____

_____

How do you feel about retailing? _____

_____

essential
5 experience *continued*

What is your philosophy about attending continuing education programs, seminars, and shows? _____

Are you willing to personally invest in your professional development? _____
_____

Describe ways in which you feel you provide excellent customer service. _____
_____

Please share some examples of consultation questions you might ask a client. _____
_____

List steps you would take to build a solid client base and ensure clients return. _____
_____

essential
experience
6

Word Scramble

Scramble	Correct Word
ticedduve gninsaoer	_ _ _ _ _ _ _ _ _ _ _ _ _ _ _ _ _ _ _ _ _ _
	Clue: Used to reach logical conclusions
loftropoi	_ _ _ _ _ _ _ _ _
	Clue: Collection of documents that reflect your skills
usemer	_ _ _ _ _ _
	Clue: Summary of education and experience
krow chiet	_ _ _ _ _ _ _ _ _
	Clue: Commitment to delivering worthy service for value received
yolpemmten	_ _ _ _ _ _ _ _ _ _
	Clue: Something you pursue after you graduate
nucomcamiinot	_ _ _ _ _ _ _ _ _ _ _ _ _
	Clue: Something needed to interact effectively with clients
trigeytin	_ _ _ _ _ _ _ _ _
	Clue: Commitment to a strong code of moral and artistic values
frenchais	_ _ _ _ _ _ _ _ _
	Clue: Having a national name and image consistent with the organization
shemtnilbatse	_ _ _ _ _ _ _ _ _ _ _ _ _
	Clue: A place where you may obtain employment
weevtiinr	_ _ _ _ _ _ _ _ _
	Clue: A meeting where your qualifications are considered

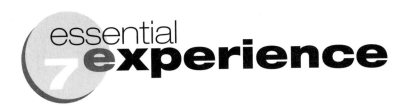

Why I Chose Cosmetology

One of the most important tasks you can complete in preparing your professional portfolio and in preparing for an effective interview is writing a brief statement about why you have chosen a career in cosmetology. In the space provided, write such a statement. Remember to include such points as an explanation of what you love about your new career; a description of your philosophy about the importance of teamwork and how you see yourself as a contributing team player; and a description of methods you would employ to increase clinic and retail revenue.

_____

_____

_____

_____

_____

_____

_____

_____

_____

_____

_____

_____

_____

_____

essential review

Using the following words, fill in the blanks below to form a thorough review of Chapter 25, "Seeking Employment." Words or terms may be used more than once.

20	broad	half million	responsibilities
30	bullheadedness	hardest	resume
50	cheating	ideals	self-confident
60	conclusions	illegal	smiling
70	contacts	integrity	solidified
80	course content	legal	speed
90	crib notes	motivation	studying
10 seconds	disinterested party	multiple choice	timing
2 minutes	documents	negative	transferable
20 seconds	down-time	network	true/false
appropriate	drawings	one million	two million
assumptions	easiest	portfolio	willpower
attention	English	practice	work ethic
autobiography	family member	qualifying	

1. Top professionals in the field of cosmetology were not born successful; they achieved success with their _____ , energy, and persistence.

2. Of all the factors that will affect your test performance on the licensing examination, the most important is your mastery of _____ .

3. A test-wise student begins to prepare for test-taking by practicing the daily habits and time management that are an important part of effective _____ .

4. On test day, it is a good idea to arrive early with a _____ attitude; be alert, calm, and ready for the challenge.

5. When taking a test, answer the _____ questions first.

6. Deductive reasoning is the process of reaching logical _____ by employing logical reasoning.

7. When applying deductive reasoning in test-taking, watch for "key" words or terms and look for _____ conditions or statements.

8. When taking a _____ test, read the entire question carefully, including all the choices.

9. An effective tip when preparing for the practical examination is to participate in "mock" licensing examinations, including the _____ of applicable examination criteria.

essential review *continued*

10. Completion of the Personal Inventory of Characteristics and Skills helps you identify any areas needing further _____ and determine where to focus the remainder of your training.

11. One key characteristic that will not only help you get the position you want, but will help you keep it, is _____ .

12. It has been determined that about _____ percent of your success will depend on your "people" skills and the remaining _____ percent will be based on your technical skills.

13. You have a strong _____ when you believe that work is good and you are committed to delivering worthy service for the value received from your employer.

14. In the United States alone, the professional salon business includes over 250,000 establishments that employ more than _____ active cosmetologists.

15. A basic value-priced salon may be a good starting place for a recent graduate because it provides for the practice of many types of haircuts, which increases self-confidence and _____ .

16. A _____ is a written summary of your education and work experience.

17. The average time a potential employer will spend scanning your resume to determine if you should be granted an interview is about _____ .

18. When writing a resume, it is more important to focus on your achievements rather than your _____ .

19. Skills which you have already mastered at other jobs that can be put to use in the new position are known as _____ .

20. An employment portfolio is a collection, usually bound, of photos and _____ that reflect your skills, accomplishments, and abilities in your chosen career field.

21. One way to determine if your portfolio portrays you and your career skills in the most positive light is to run it by a _____ for feedback and suggestions about how to make it more interesting and accurate.

22. When visiting salons prior to requesting an employment interview, remember that it is important to never burn your bridges, but rather build a _____ of contacts who have a favorable opinion of you.

23. _____ is the universal language.

24. On an employment application, questions regarding race, religion, or national origin are considered to be _____ .

25. Once you have obtained that important first job, remember that how you use _____ can be critical in ensuring your future success on the job.

essential
discoveries and
accomplishments

In the space below, jot some notes about what concepts of this chapter were hardest for you to understand or remember. Imagine finding yourself suddenly in the role of "teacher" and consider what you would tell your "students" about these difficult concepts.

Share your *Essential Discoveries* with some of the other students in your class and ask if they are helpful to them. You may want to revise your notes based on good ideas shared by your peers. Under "Accomplishments," list at least three things you have accomplished since your last entry that relate to your career goals.

Discoveries:

_____

_____

_____

_____

_____

Accomplishments:

_____

_____

_____

_____

_____

On The Job

After studying this chapter and completing the Essential
Companion *components, you should be able to:*

1. Describe the qualities that help a new employee succeed in a service profession.

2. List the habits of a good salon team player.

3. Explain the function of a job description.

4. Describe three different ways in which salon professionals are compensated.

5. Create a personal budget.

6. List the principles of selling products and services in the salon.

7. List the most effective ways to build a client base.

essential
on the job
satisfaction

Why do I need to learn about making the transition from school to work?

It has been said that as much as 80 percent of your career success will result from personal attributes such as your people skills, your ability to communicate, your visual integrity, and your goal orientations. If only 20 percent of your career success has to do with your technical skills, it stands to reason that there are many more qualities you need to work on to achieve that desired level of success. The cosmetologists who achieve that goal stay with the profession longer than the rest, own or work in successful salons, and enjoy all the rewards of success. They all started out with stars in their eyes. However, they knew it took more than just a dream. They knew it would take commitment and hard work, and they made sure they were prepared for every opportunity that came knocking.

As professionals-in-training they came to school early and stayed late as needed. They accepted those late clients without whining. They wrapped and rewrapped those design texture services on mannequin after mannequin to ensure quality and competitive speed. They read industry journals and stayed abreast of the daily changes happening within the field of cosmetology. The important thing to remember here is that these professionals-in-training became full-fledged, licensed professionals.

If you consider yourself among this elite class, you know that you were not born but rather made yourself into who you are today by your own desires, energies, and persistence. You recognize that being a stylist is not a 9-to-5 job 4 days a week. It's being there whenever your clients need you. You know that it's going the extra mile, taking the extra client, and biting back those angry words that spring up when a client is rude or a coworker is unfair. It's paying your dues, mastering your craft, building self-confidence, and developing a strong personal pride in your accomplishments.

Tis easy enough to be pleasant when life flows like a song, but the man worthwhile is the one who will smile when everything goes dead wrong.
—Ella Wheeler Wilcox

essential concepts of satisfaction on the job

What do I need to know about making the transition from school to work in order to maintain satisfaction and success on the job?

While you are probably very excited about having your first paying job in your new career, there are a number of responsibilities that go along with that paycheck. Your school environment has been a relatively safe and comfortable one. Here, you have had the opportunity to practice service after service to get to the desired results. On the job, your clients will expect the desired results the first time around. In school you have had to deal with the institution's tardy policy, which was probably quite lenient compared to that of the salon. Clients are not very forgiving when you are not at work at the appointed time to provide their service.

While in school you probably had more flexibility in dealing with your personal schedule as it related to your class schedule. On the job you will be expected to be at work every day as scheduled, promptly, and ready to work when you arrive. At school you may have had the opportunity to do your hair or your makeup after you clocked in . . . which is not the case in the workplace. If you just didn't feel like going to school on any given day, perhaps you just didn't go. A job with a paycheck brings with it an expectation of more maturity than that.

Therefore, you need to realize that, on the job, you are responsible for many more decisions and for performing in a professional manner at all times, even when you do not feel like it. On the job you will need to be focused on constantly building a business rather than watching the clock to see how long it is until your required hours have been clocked. In addition, you will need to concentrate on furthering your knowledge and skills to remain abreast of all the new trends, tools, and techniques your new job presents. All in all, it's an exciting new opportunity, one that has many rewards accompanied by many responsibilities.

essential
experience
1

Evaluate Your Skills—Are You Job Ready?

Take a few minutes to think back over your training and your clinic experience and reflect on all you have learned that you didn't know when you started. Give yourself a hearty pat on the back for your accomplishments. Then evaluate your skills and check those in which you feel confident. If you need more practice, indicate that by checking that column. Then make a personal commitment to improvement in those areas.

Subject Area	Competent	Need Improvement
Infection control		
Product knowledge		
Hair chemistry		
Shampooing		
Haircutting		
Blunt shapes		
Graduated shapes		
Layered shapes		
Clipper cutting		
Other cutting techniques		
Hair texturizing		
Texture services		
Relaxer services		
Mixing solutions		
Wrapping		
Processing		
Haircoloring		
Color wheel		
Levels of color		
Brush application		
One process		
Two process		
Retouch		
Foil highlights		
Mixing color (tube and liquid)		

Subject Area	Competent	Need Improvement
Style finishing		
Blow-dry		
Round brush		
Curling iron		
Wet sets		
Styling aids		
Client communications		
Eye contact		
Handshake		
Open-ended questions		
Active listening		
Developing rapport		
Client consultation		
Greeting		
Analysis		
Recommendations		
Client record keeping		
Client development		
Client retention		
Client referrals		
Client rebooking		
Retail product sales		
Ticket upgrading		
Salon/clinic teamwork		
Work ethic		
Productivity		
Receptionist duties		
Industry knowledge		
Time management		
Goal setting		
Personal finances		
Job hunting skills		
Career planning		

essential
2 experience

Technical Skills Improvement

Based on the analysis you completed in Essential Experience #1, create a plan of action for every area you checked as needing improvement. Record your plan in the space provided.

_____

_____

_____

_____

_____

_____

_____

_____

_____

_____

_____

_____

_____

_____

_____

_____

_____

_____

essential
3 experience

Career Management

In today's market there are more jobs available than there are stylists to fill them. Thus, you owe it to yourself, and your potential new employer, to find the best fit possible. Once you have made that decision, stick with it and give it your absolute best as long as you can. Job hopping early in your career is not good for your professional development or your reputation. Following are several pointers that will help you right from the start. In the column to the right of the pointers, explain how you intend to make the most of each suggestion.

Pointer	Plan of Action
Master the techniques you learned in Chapter 25 to ensure you find the right job for your strengths and preferences.	
Understand that your income grows when you work harder, build a sound client base, volunteer for extra clients, sell retail, and show initiative and ambition.	
Arrive for work at least 15 minutes prior to your first client, dressed and groomed, ready to work.	
Have your station set up and ready for each scheduled service before the client arrives.	
Know that your clients and the salon are relying on you to be there. Only call in sick if you are absolutely sick.	
Have realistic expectations of how much money you will earn your first year. It takes time to build a loyal client base.	
Build a realistic personal budget and stick to it. Don't spend more than you make!	
Continue to study, train, and expand your personal and your technical skills.	
Join your local cosmetology association and attend meetings faithfully.	

essential
4 experience

Planning Your Future

You are about to complete a major step in your journey toward career success: graduation from cosmetology school. Now it's time to think about building a client base for the future. If you have already targeted area salons and secured a position in one of them, it is appropriate to begin building a client base to join you there.

Create a client development list. These are people you would like to contact about trying your services. Determine how many clients you would like to have when you begin your new job. Create a plan with a goal of contacting a certain number of people every week for at least one month. Give these contacts your new place of employment and schedule them for an appointment.

After you get into the salon and perform the services, follow up each salon visit with a phone call and ask about the service you provided. Make sure the client is still satisfied and find out if there is anything else you can do. If possible, rebook your clients for a future service.

Use the following space to list the potential clients you want to contact.

NAME   PHONE NUMBER

_____

_____

_____

_____

_____

_____

_____

essential
5 experience

Teamwork

As a contributing team member in the salon, you will be called upon to deal with a variety of problems or situations on a regular basis. In order to build your teamwork skills while you are in school, work with a couple of other classmates. Consider the following situations and how you would handle them in the workplace. Record your results in the space provided.

1. You each arrive for work with a fully booked schedule for the day. The manager and two other stylists have been stricken with the flu and will not make it into work today. You and your teammates have to decide how to handle the clients of the other three stylists. What do you do?

    _____

    _____

    _____

    _____

2. Your salon owner is remodeling the facility, which includes reorganizing the space and assigning new work stations to everyone. You and your classmates are to discuss and develop some criteria the owner could use in assigning new stations since some of the spaces are more desirable than others.

    _____

    _____

    _____

    _____

3. The salon's manager states the plan of implementing a retail bonus plan for all stylists and asks for your help in developing the policy. You and your classmates are to create a retail bonus plan that you would recommend for adoption.

    _____

    _____

    _____

    _____

essential
6 experience

The Job Description

Assume you are the owner of a highly successful salon. Write a job description for a junior stylist listing all the factors you deem appropriate to the position.

_____

_____

_____

_____

_____

_____

_____

_____

_____

_____

_____

_____

_____

_____

_____

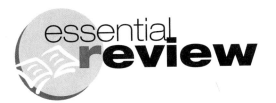

Using the following words, fill in the blanks below to form a thorough review of Chapter 26, "On The Job." Words may be used more than once or not at all.

client consultations	feelings or desires	job description	retailing
commissions	financial	mathematical	salary
compensation	grateful	mature	serving
conflict	immature	pay raise	temptations
doubt	increasing	resolution	ticket upgrading
educational	issues	respectful	

1. When seeking your first salon job, it is important to ask yourself some key questions such as what your _____ goals are.

2. Another personal consideration when looking for your first job is to think about what _____ you care most deeply about.

3. The number one thing to remember when you are in a service business is that your work revolves around _____ your clients.

4. In the salon you will have to quickly get used to putting your own _____ aside and putting the needs of the salon and the client first.

5. Getting to work on time is _____ not only to your clients but also to your coworkers who will have to handle your clients if you are late.

6. Remember that it is an honor to have a job that will provide you and your family with financial stability, so be very _____.

7. Although you may not like or agree with the salon manager or her rules, you must give her the benefit of the _____.

8. Thinking that you will never need to learn anything more once you are out of school is _____ and limiting.

9. Given the stress of a typical salon, there will be lots of opportunities for you to become negative or to have conflicts with your teammates. Resist the _____ to give in to maliciousness and gossip.

10. The most difficult part of being in a relationship, whether it is a personal or professional relationship, is when _____ arises.

essential review *continued*

11. When assuming a new position, you are agreeing to do everything as it is written down in a _____, so if you are unclear about something or need more information, it is your responsibility to ask.

12. Being paid a flat rate of the same amount of dollars no matter how many hours you actually work is known as being paid a _____ .

13. _____ are paid on percentages of your total service dollars and can range anywhere from 25 percent to 70 percent, depending on your length of time at the salon and your performance levels.

14. When deciding whether a certain _____ method is right for you, it is important to be aware of what your monthly expenses are and to have a personal financial budget and plan in place.

15. Ask a senior stylist to sit in on one of your _____ and to make note of areas where you can improve.

16. Although a career in the beauty industry is very artistic and creative, it is also a career that requires _____ understanding and planning.

17. Many people are afraid of the word "budget" because they think it will be too restrictive on their spending or because they think they need to be _____ geniuses in order to work with a budget.

18. You will want to think about other ways to increase your income including spending less money and _____ service prices.

19. _____ or upselling services is the practice of recommending and selling additional services to your clients, which may be performed by you or by other practitioners in the salon.

20. _____ is the act of recommending and selling products to your clients for at-home hair, skin, and nail care.

essential discoveries and accomplishments

In the space below, jot some notes about what concepts of this chapter were hardest for you to understand or remember. Imagine finding yourself suddenly in the role of "teacher" and consider what you would tell your "students" about these difficult concepts.

Share your **Essential Discoveries** with some of the other students in your class and ask if they are helpful to them. You may want to revise your notes based on good ideas shared by your peers. Under "Accomplishments," list at least three things you have accomplished since your last entry that relate to your career goals.

Discoveries:

_____

_____

_____

_____

_____

Accomplishments:

_____

_____

_____

_____

_____